A TRANSFORMATIONAL THEORY OF AESTHETICS

How we perceive and respond to the visual image has been a traditional concern of psychologists, philosophers and art historians. Today, where the visual image increasingly permeates our everyday life and consciousness, the question becomes ever more relevant. How do we, for instance, instinctively 'know'what it is that a picture represents without having to be taught? How is it that we experience (aesthetic) pleasure in looking at certain pictures? How is it that we often want to talk about the pictures we look at?

Such questions are currently asked by a wide range of disciplines, including: semiotics, psychoanalysis, anthropology, neuropsychology, and in general, contemporary critical analysis of the visual arts.

In *A Transformational Theory of Aesthetics*, Michael Stephan breaks new ground by linking the findings of these areas. Drawing on their common area of knowledge, he has developed a radically new theory of picture perception and aesthetic response, arguing that images can generate in us a complex pattern of mental changes, or transformations. This is because the left and right hemispheres of the brain do not always work in harmony, hence the wide-ranging nature of aesthetic response to distinct art forms.

A Transformational Theory of Aesthetics is essential reading to those seriously involved in linking the arts and cognitive sciences.

THE AUTHOR

Michael Stephan was born in 1948 in St Helier, Jersey. He currently lectures in the University of London and completed his doctoral research in the University of Sussex. He was a postgraduate Fine Art student at the Slade School, University College, London and has exhibited his work widely in Britain and Europe.

A TRANSFORMATIONAL THEORY OF AESTHETICS

MICHAEL STEPHAN

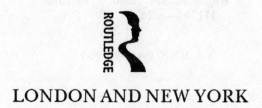

LONDON AND NEW YORK

First published 1990
by Routledge
11 New Fetter Lane, London EC4P 4EE

Simultaneously published in the USA and Canada
by Routledge
a division of Routledge, Chapman and Hall, Inc.
29 West 35th Street, New York, NY 10001

© 1990 Michael Stephan

Typeset by NWL Editorial Services
Langport, Somerset TA10 9DG

Printed and bound in Great Britain by Mackays of Chatham

British Library Cataloguing in Publication Data
Stephan, Michael, *1948 –*
A transformational theory of aesthetics
1. Visual perception
I. Title
152.1'4

Library of Congress Cataloging in Publication Data
Stephan, Michael, 1948 –
A transformational theory of aesthetics / by Michael Stephan.
p.   cm.
Includes bibliographical references.
1. Aesthetics–Psychological aspects.   I. Title.
BH301.P45S74   1990   89–70164
111'.85—dc20   CIP

ISBN 0-415-04196-1

FOR HEATHER AND LAURENCE

CONTENTS

vii

FIGURES

FOREWORD

Trevor Pateman

We are all in favour of interdisciplinary work, just as we are all in favour of virtue. But in practice we are often sinners, and intellectual inhibition, not to mention the restrictive practices of academic guilds, ensures that little enough interdisciplinary work is actually done. When it is, the business of peer review often breaks down because there are not enough peers about with the competence or confidence to engage with its challenges.

Despite such hazards Michael Stephan has acted boldly. In this book he does this by thinking through the medium of an extensive literature in neuropsychology, cognitive science, psychoanalysis, aesthetics, and art history – a particular combination of sources with which it is unlikely that anyone else has completely engaged. He speculates freely and offers us a bold theorization of our immediate experience of, and reflexive relationship to, representational imagery and, in particular, painting.

His approach is carefully naturalistic; not for him the vapourings of those who plague us with Real Presences. He uses the findings of contemporary neuropsychology, and especially work on hemispheric lateralization of cognitive function, to build a theory which shows that the answers to some of the apparently disparate questions we ask about picture perception are, in fact, interconnected.

Consider five such questions. (1) How is it that we can, in general, recognize what a picture is a picture of without instruction in the principles or conventions according to which it is constructed? (2) How is it that children's drawings change in the developmental sequence they do? (3) How is it that we experience (aesthetic) pleasure in looking at (some) pictures? (4) How do we reconcile the idea that we get 'involved' with a work of art with the idea that aesthetic experience involves keeping some kind of 'psychical distance'? (5) How is it that, so often, we want to talk about the pictures we look at?

In Michael Stephan's account, answers to these apparently disconnected questions fall out in an orderly, connected fashion from the theory he develops. That is, I think, a remarkable achievement.

Here is not the place to summarize Stephan's theory. You must read the book to find out what it is. Let me just remark on an aspect and a consequence of his work.

Stephan resists the contemporary tendency, often inspired by practical considerations, to assimilate the arts and to treat aesthetic experience as undifferentiated with respect to the different arts. If parts of the brain and mind are as specialized in their structure and function as neuroscientists and cognitive psychologists tell us, it would indeed be surprising if 'the arts' or 'aesthetic experience' formed a natural kind. Stephan positively suggests that they do not. His canvas is broad, but it has a well-defined edge: he claims only to account for our experience of representational images.

In doing so, he does, however, blur or eliminate the distinction between the character of our experience of paintings and photographs – a distinction on which many writers (Roger Scruton, for example) have insisted. This is so because Stephan insists that in looking at a painting, extensive networks of recognitory memory are unconsciously and non-introspectibly activated, and enter into our experience of the painting in ways similar or identical to the way in which the sense of the having-been-there of a real object enters into our experience of looking at a photograph. Of course, distinctions between paintings and photographs remain, but if Stephan is right, paintings and photographs are not so different as some of us (I include myself) have wanted to think.

Unfortunately, this is not the place for an essay on that subject. It remains for me to say that I have been provoked to many thoughts during the years of my association with Michael Stephan's work. I very much hope that other readers are also provoked to thoughts of their own as they proceed to the text – but that before they do that, they will note, in passing, the institutional location of the less than usually restrictive academic guild which allowed his work to be completed.

Trevor Pateman
Institute of Continuing and Professional Education
University of Sussex   July 1989

INTRODUCTION

1 GENERAL

The views advanced in this book draw from several disciplines on the assumption that each shares a common area of knowledge which, if synthesized, is capable of leading to a new paradigm applicable to contemporary critical analysis of the visual arts and in particular to theories of picture perception and aesthetic response. It therefore follows in the tradition favoured by Gombrich and being developed by the Harvard Project Zero collaboration.[1] This tradition believes it is precisely in the course of interdisciplinary probings into the arts that significant insights into its nature and implications are likely to be discovered.

More particularly, if we favour the view that certain issues of concern to contemporary psychology are relevant, this supposes that our relations to the arts can be understood in terms of cognition, for the present best defined as the *act of knowing*, with the implication that different art forms suppose distinct *ways* of knowing. Differentiating the arts in these terms suggests that the way of knowing pertaining to the visual arts can be distinguished from the one pertaining to music, literature, or any of the other arts. This has as a possible corollary that aspects of our mental life are specialized and distinct ways of knowing are neither necessarily compatible nor inter-translatable.

2 THE TRANSLATION AND CAUSATION ISSUES

The question of 'translatability' raises an epistemological issue central to the visual arts. This is that difficulties are bound to arise when the art theoretician, whose communicative mode lies in the manipulation of a linguistically structured symbol system, attempts to explicate the work of the artist whose mode lies in the manipulation of a visually structured one.[2] Given that we live in a linguistically dominated culture, the implication is that language could easily be applied in accordance with its distinct way of knowing to encourage limited formulations of the visual arts while inhibiting other formulations. This would not be difficult given language's facility as an arbitrary and discursive sign to abstract and conceptualize our experience of the world.

But here it should be emphasized that the use of language to abstract and conceptualize is not meant as a criticism, given that the language capacity is rightly considered one of the major features which distinguish us as a species. What is questionable, from a cognitively underpinned viewpoint, is the extent to which language can plausibly explicate the visual image (the translation issue) and, if it cannot, what is it which, regardless, continues to motivate its use by all visual art related hermeneutic disciplines (the causation issue)? These are important (although I believe much neglected) questions, if we are of the view that our capacity to produce visual art also distinguishes us as a species, with the implication that its form constitutes an evolved communication system in its own right not requiring linguistic intervention to explain its meaning.[3] In fact, it can be argued that the whole purpose of the visual image is to present us with an *iconic* (Peirce 1940) reminder of our experience of the world thereby eliciting its unique (non-linguistic) way of knowing.

At least two assumptions have just been implied that require brief clarification because of their centrality to my conclusions. First, that our perceptions of the representational visual image do not require training in a convention (we do not need to *learn* to see pictures), thereby indicating that representations are universally (cross-culturally) recognizable for innately determined reasons. Second, that our perceptions occur relative to an extra-visually as well as visually constituted memory system, thereby accounting for an image's capacity to elicit experientially derived knowledge of a general kind (cf. Wollheim 1987: 100).

In the first instance, my view is that we understand the representational visual image because the nature of the light reflected from its surface sensibly corresponds, in certain essential respects, to how we habitually perceive the phenomenal world. From this it follows that our understanding is something akin to a reflex action, that is, the juxtaposed visual elements constituting the image automatically 'trigger' our knowledge of what it represents (cf. Kennedy 1974, 1977; Marr 1982).

In the second instance, if our perceptions did not include reference to a complex (a typically extra- as well as visually derived) memory system, then an image would never rise above visual abstraction. That is, by definition, a *re*presentation is surely a reminder of something known and therefore necessarily experienced in general form. (I return to the implications of these views in section 6 of this introduction.)

For the present it can be noted that the translation issue is not new to the visual arts. Gombrich, for example, sees it as constituting a 'notorious difficulty' and freely admits that the unique character of personal (visual) expression makes it quite untranslatable into words. The difficulty has less to do with art than with language, however, because, 'Neither a real apple nor one by Cézanne can ever be exhaustively described for the simple reason that the variety of apples are infinite but the number of words in any language is strictly finite' (1978: 100).[4]

Having proposed that the representational visual image can never be effectively explicated through recourse to the linguistic sign, Gombrich thereafter shifts his hermeneutic ground by proposing that, in fact, the art theoretician's task should be to find clear and unambiguous linguistic terms for each of the possibilities the artist rejected or selected. Because these terms cannot be at hand in everyday life, however, the best the theoretician can hope for, 'is to search for equivalent gamuts that allow him to convey his meaning through metaphor and analogy' (100).

In this way Gombrich unsuccessfully attempts to avoid his own 'notorious difficulty' (of translation) by entering into areas even more epistemologically problematic. That is, having maintained that the representational image is untranslatable into words, he nonetheless assumes that certain (intentional) aspects of artistic activity (the possibilities the artist rejected or selected) can be unambiguously interpreted through metaphor and analogy. The logical inference is that art theoreticians are capable of reading artists' minds through the vehicle of their work and are thereafter capable of conveying their findings through a much debated branch of language study.

At this point we are surely entitled to ask: are Gombrich's equivalent (linguistic) gamuts truly equivalents or do they constitute a semantically autonomous sign system capable of forming nothing more than a lengthy *anchorage* to direct or misdirect, as the case may be, our perceptions of the representational image?[5] This question has important implications when it is considered that a theoretician of Panofsky's status insists that a true appreciation of representational art is contingent upon iconographical analysis, a form which presupposes a familiarity with specific themes or concepts transmitted through literary sources, whether acquired by purposeful reading or oral tradition (Panofsky 1955). Yet surely few would argue that a true appreciation of literature is contingent upon a familiarity with specific themes or concepts transmitted through visual means?

3 NON-INTROSPECTIBILITY AND THE VISUAL ARTS

We have only just entered the epistemological labyrinth, that is, scepticism regarding the grounds for supposing that different symbol systems are inter-translatable and therefore 'inter-knowable'. This is because many of the ways of knowing pertaining to the visual arts are often considered to be non-introspectible and we are therefore entitled to be ontologically sceptical about the nature of their existence (cf. Pateman 1985). Perkins and Leondar also refer to this dimension when they propose that, 'Generally we proceed unaware of the busy-work involved in perceiving because much of it proceeds rapidly and non-consciously' (1977: 3).[6]

If aspects of cognition pertaining to the visual arts are considered to be non-introspectible, however, the art theoretician has every right to ask: What grounds exist for supposing that, *mutatis mutandis*, the use of language, albeit an imperfect form, is at least not the best possible way to explicate the meaning of art? Contrarily, if the character of the (assumed) non-introspectible in art can be elucidated, the corollary assumption is that implications can be drawn regarding whether its meaning can or cannot (and therefore should or should not) be properly communicated through linguistic agencies. If the conclusion is that it cannot, then we are surely entitled to challenge proposals à la Panofsky and press the question: what is it which motivates their construction?

Although I pretend no simple solutions to how a greater understanding of the non-introspectible in art can be achieved, a clue surely lies in examining its definition, taking into account once again our linguistically dominated culture. That is, is the non-introspectible generally conceived of as denoting something not readily available to that way of knowing readily formulated and communicated through a *linguistically* structured symbol system? If this is the case, and it is conceded that non-discursive but intuitive ways of knowing are relevant to introspection, then Perkins and Leondar are right when they propose that 'Cognition, or "knowing" is too easily construed as solely a matter of words and their silent manipulation' (1977: 2). Simply recognizing this proposition shifts the emphasis from aspects of cognition being non-introspectible (with the connotation that they are forever out of reach) to them being simply unavailable to forms of linguistically underpinned consciousness. This has as a possible corollary that if the correct strategy is employed they can become the object of serious study thereby contributing to our greater understanding of the visual arts.

4 A NEUROPSYCHOLOGICAL PERSPECTIVE OF THE NON-DISCURSIVE

There are perhaps several ways to approach the non-discursive in art. The one I have favoured is to refer primarily to the neuropsychological evidence and in particular to the clinical data resulting from lateralization research.

Given that the human brain is universal and it follows that a greater understanding of its function is relevant to common areas of human activity, referring to this type of knowledge is a sound research strategy for a number of reasons. To begin with, because neuropsychology is interested in the relations between the brain and what it produces, its evidence is biologically substantiated and to that extent relatively empirical. More specifically in relation to gaining a greater understanding of the meaning of art, by studying the brain damaged and paying particular attention to the role played in cognition by the right 'non-discursive' hemisphere, neuropsychology has illuminated many ordinary competences normally considered unavailable to serious study, as Pateman indicates.

Faculty psychology underpinned by the findings of brain researchers like A.R. Luria (*The Man with the Shattered World*) and Michael Gazzaniga and Roger Sperry (right and left hemisphere specialization) makes very good sense of what we know about human potential. And using the extraordinary cases of brain damage and prodigious talent to illuminate the structure of ordinary competences is a sound research strategy: the disabled and the abled are, for the scientist, naturally occurring experiments.

(Pateman 1984a: 28)

Many instances of such naturally occurring experiments and their implications are related in this book, but for the present the mental competences associated with the right hemisphere and their relevance to the non-discursive in visual art, is best encapsulated by referring to Sperry's Nobel Prize speech.

It proved possible to demonstrate further that the so-called subordinate or minor hemisphere, which we had formerly supposed to be illiterate and mentally retarded and thought by some authorities not even to be conscious, was found to be the superior or cerebral member when it came to performing certain kinds of mental tasks. The right-hemisphere specialities were all, of course, nonverbal, nonmathematical, and nonsequential. They were largely spatial and imagistic, the kind in which a single picture or mental image is worth a thousand words.

(Sperry 1982: 1224–5)

Sperry later confirms this view and adds:

The left and right hemispheres of the brain are each found to have their own specialized forms of intellect. The left is highly verbal and mathematical, and performs with analytic, symbolic, computer-like sequential logic. The right, by contrast, is spatial, mute, and performs with a synthetic, spatioperceptual and mechanical kind of processing not yet simulatable in computers.

(Sperry 1983: 56)

I should emphasize that the exact cerebral localization of function is not in itself central to my arguments, however. What is relevant is that lateralization research has established that non-discursive ways of knowing have a clear biological and evolutionary foundation. Equally relevant are the indications that certain non-discursive mental competences relevant to the meaning of art are capable of successfully functioning without direct linguistic intervention.

The importance of establishing a biological and evolutionary foundation for non-discursive mental competences and their possible relations to art becomes all the more relevant when it is considered that, until comparatively recently, very little was known about either the corpus callosum, which allows information to pass between the hemispheres, or the right cerebral hemisphere.[7] Only since the early 1960s has brain research concentrated on substantiating the role played in cognition by one entire half of the human cortex. The point here is, although neither the corpus callosum nor the right hemisphere phylogenetically developed overnight, it is a reasonable assumption that the lack of emphasis given, until recently, to the right hemisphere was indicative of an ideological indifference in recognizing the role non-discursive ways of knowing play in processing information.[8]

This view is substantiated by the neuropsychologists Gazzaniga and LeDoux's proposal, 'The memory mechanism that psychologists have been studying *ad nauseam*, is the verbal processing system' (1978: 135). They continue by arguing however: what if all the memory systems are not equally available to that way of knowing associated with our language and speech systems (a specific way of introspecting) and linguistically resistant ways of knowing suppose their own modes of response? If this is recognized, then:

> The name of the game becomes quite different. Now the non-verbal systems have an opportunity to express themselves by pointing to a series of objects, and with this response possible, all the information that the multiple, nonverbal systems have stored can be reported, making the entire system more resourceful.
>
> (Gazzaniga and LeDoux 1978: 136)[9]

The researchers are referring to the classic distinction between recognition and recall and attributing them an equal (cognitive) status. From this follows their emphasis that when the nonverbal systems have an equal opportunity to express themselves the entire system becomes more resourceful. Because picture perception relies heavily upon the recognitory memory system, Gazzaniga and

7

LeDoux's views are referred to at some length in this book. For the present it suffices to say that any account of human behaviour obscuring the significance of linguistically resistant modes of understanding and response from its dialogue will surely be an impoverished one.

5 THE COMPATIBILITY PROPOSITION

If the respective hemispheres possess qualitatively different modes of cognitive processing it is a reasonable assumption that these developed for some good evolutionary reasons which carry over, as it were, to affect the way in which symbol systems and information generally found in the culture are processed. From this it follows that certain symbolic stimuli forms are more likely to elicit, and therefore be compatible with, certain modes of cognitive processing while inhibiting others. This essentially modular view of cerebral development suggests the following possibility.

Our evolved capacity to automatically understand iconic symbol forms – pictures, for example – is closely associated with the same mental paradigm which evolved to allow our species to readily perceive visually and subsequently respond to the three- dimensional world.[10] This capacity must have been necessary to prehistorical humans for purely practical reasons – instantly recognizing and avoiding dangerous animals, for example. Similarly, our evolved capacity to translate arbitrary symbol forms – syntax, for example – is closely associated with the same mental paradigm which evolved to allow our species to abstract information from the world thereby facilitating its (cognitive) manipulation in its phenomenal absence. This capacity must have afforded prehistorical humans the distinct advantage of being able to plan their actions.

This hypothesis concurs in general with Marr's *principle of modular design* which states that evolutionary changes occurring in one part of the brain need not have been accompanied by simultaneous compensatory changes elsewhere. Therefore, taking into account lateralization research, changes that occurred in the left hemisphere (around the classical language centres of Broca and Wernicke, for example) to affect its processing mode, need not have occurred in the right hemisphere; thereafter, changes that occurred in the right hemisphere (around the right parietal lobe, for example) to affect its processing mode need not have occurred in the left, and so forth (cf. Broca 1861; Warrington and Taylor 1973, 1978; Levy 1969, 1974; Marr 1982).

If the brain evolved different modes of cognitive processing that are activated by distinct symbol forms, then it surely follows that Gombrich's 'notorious difficulty' (of translation) is cerebrally endogenous. That is, we are talking about the problem of, at a minimum, two distinct neuropsychologically defined 'ways of knowing' competing to process a common stimuli form, namely, the representational visual image.

Given my compatibility proposition, it follows that the intervention of (left-hemisphere associated) linguistically structured ways of knowing to explicate the visual image (a right-hemisphere associated way of knowing) can be seen as often being simply misplaced. That is, our perceptions of conventional and iconic symbol forms (language and pictures, for example) elicit distinct modes of cognitive processing that are neither readily inter-translatable nor 'inter-knowable'.

It is therefore not so much a case of a picture being worth a thousand words, as proposed by Sperry, or a thousand words being worth a picture – rather, it is a case of it being questionable, on evolutionary and neuropsychological grounds, to expect any amount of words to explicate a picture or vice versa.

This has as a possible corollary that there are good reasons for supposing that the intention to verbally explicate at least certain forms of visual imagery is a symptom of left (language) hemisphere dominance and more generally an ideological reflection of culture's tendency to celebrate exclusively linguistic ways of knowing.

Linguistic dominance in general is perhaps most easily accounted for by noting the inherent communicative natures of the respective symbol forms involved in my contention, namely, language and visual imagery. Consequently, because language is discursive it has the potential to explicate the visual image, whereas because visual imagery is an essentially non-discursive symbol form, it does not possess the same facility in regard to language. In other words, the hermeneutical flow is unidirectional.

I have so far referred to some of the major themes and views developed over the following chapters. My conclusions lead me to propose that the tendency to verbalize the visual, and in particular the representational visual image, is not solely a result of linguistic dominance per se, however, but is also linked to the anomalous position the representational image occupies in our psychology, as I shall now attempt to briefly show.

6 THE REPRESENTATIONAL VISUAL IMAGE

I have introduced the argument that our capacity to understand iconic symbol forms is associated with the same right-hemisphere associated mental paradigm which evolved, for purely practical reasons, to enable our species to cope with the vicissitudes of the phenomenal world. This leads me to hypothesize that a greater understanding of the causation and translation issues necessarily benefits from including the phenomenal world as the third term in the relationship proposed in schema 1.

Schema 1

phenomenal world → its iconic representation → the latter's linguistic representation

My reasoning is that if we take into account the nature of our existential relations to phenomena, this should help to illuminate the nature of our subsequent relations to its iconic *re*presentation.

Our existential relations to phenomena are clearly complex but from a developmental perspective include what Piaget (1966) terms *intersensorial perception*. That is, the fact that information often reaches our higher cognitive systems after being relayed via two or more sense modalities, thereby affording us a comprehensive or *maximum grasp* understanding of the nature of the world (cf. Merleau Ponty 1962; Dreyfus 1972; Fodor 1983).

Something as mundane as fruit, for example, may be (intersensorially) perceived and identified through all five sense modalities. On seeing an apple (sight) we may pick it up (touch) and proceed to eat it, thereby experiencing its particular taste, smell, and the sound it produces on being eaten. Intersensorial perception has the implication that from early childhood the way in which phenomena are sensibly mediated encodes in us certain expectations and response tendencies. That is, on seeing an apple we expect it to exhibit certain extra-visual as well as visually derived characteristics of the kind just exampled.

Given that our existential relations to the world developmentally and psychologically precede and affect our perceptions of its iconic representation, then there exist substantial grounds for supposing that pictures are perceived and responded to in terms of more than their potential simply to visually represent the world. That is, as iconic representations of a typically intersensorially perceived world, pictures contain the potential to elicit traces of our extra- as well as visually derived knowledge (with certain possible cognitive and behavioural consequences, as we shall see in a moment).

Pictures are not, therefore, perceived in visual isolation, disembodied from the world to which they refer, but are possessed of what I come to term a *full existential life*. It is, however, a life that is not readily linguistically introspectible because of its origins in the right-hemisphere 'non-discursive' cognitive paradigm. This conclusion leads me to construct a hypothesis as to why certain representational visual images, and in particular the art image, are not only habitually verbalized but also associated with a certain kind of aesthetic experience. I have termed this hypothesis a *transformational theory of aesthetics*.

7   A TRANSFORMATIONAL THEORY OF AESTHETICS

While aesthetic experience may constitute the core of aesthetics, a consensus as to its precise nature does not exist (cf. Hospers 1976). Nonetheless, probably a majority of aestheticians view the experience as being of a special kind and often related to our experience of works of visual art. This confinement does not simplify matters, however, because it raises the traditional and enormous question, what is art? This is not a question I wish to go into here but it can be noted that the possible nature of the relations between art and aesthetic experience are addressed in chapter 8.

For the present it is sufficient to say that I have developed a theory of aesthetic response which, to the best of my knowledge, is the first to be constructed taking into account the neuropsychological data.[11] It proposes that our initially right-hemisphere associated visual perceptions of the representational visual image can cause a series of essentially adaptive cognitive transformations which result in a special kind of experience.

Central to my theory is the view I have indicated, namely, that visual images are not initially perceived in visual isolation but have the potential for a full existential life. Further, if it sufficiently involves us, this life can activate phenomenally derived associations, expectations and response tendencies. Clearly, however, any such expectations and response tendencies cannot be sensibly accommodated because of an image's material constraints. We can no more manually examine the forms visually suggested by a still-life than we can corporeally enter into sexual relations with visual erotica.

In virtue of their illusory three-dimensionality, therefore, certain marks on a surface *psychologically* suggest our involved visual-spatial and existentially-derived understanding of the phenomenal world, yet their *phenomenal* two-dimensionality ensures that they necessarily remain distinctly apart from it. In this way the representational image proposes a perceptual paradox, existing as it does in what I come to term an *equivocal reality*.

These conclusions lead me to contend that an image's (material) inability to resolve certain associations, expectations, and response tendencies, can result in a subtle state of emotional arousal in the percipient.[12] This state subsequently produces emotional tensions which seek completion or resolution through some form of emotional outlet (this outlet having the function of releasing and dissipating the tensions). In this regard I refer to the views of George Mandler (1975).

Given that there typically exist no overt ways of releasing such tensions, however, it could appear that the percipient is faced with a tension-ridden and circular 'cognitive impasse'. That is, any tensions generated by our perceptions of the representational visual image could in principle continue *ad infinitum*, or at least for the duration of its perception.

I continue by hypothesizing, however, that it is eventually the image itself which (paradoxically) offers a form of emotional release, a way of (vicariously) resolving the expectations, responses, and subsequent emotional tensions it activates in virtue of its existential connotations. Thus, with all possible forms of emotional release effectively 'blocked', it has to be effected through some form of paradigm shift or psychological change on our part. This is done by a concentrated projection or what I term a *cathectic transference* of the emotional tensions 'into' the one relevant outlet readily available to perception, the representational image itself. This transference has the subsequent and significant effect of (psychologically) transforming the representation (in the eye of the beholder) into appearing to become (extraordinarily) psychologically energized, into appearing to possess what I term as *affective import*.

Although affective import is a primarily right-hemisphere generated and non-discursive phenomenon, however, it is communicated in holistic form to the left hemisphere, and in particular to its language centres, where it is discursively accommodated. This accommodation can result in affective import becoming (discursively) associated with a certain kind of aesthetic experience and the image which appears to generate it being identified as the object of aesthetic experience.

Because the (left-hemisphere associated) language centres possess no direct knowledge of the causes of this experience due to its association with right-hemisphere (non-discursive) modes of processing, however, this has typically resulted in a consensus that it is an elusive and enigmatic phenomenon. Nonetheless, by and large, this enigma is not accepted but on the contrary often forms the basis for a variety of both traditional and contemporary dialogues on the nature of aesthetic experience and its associated object, for my purposes the representational visual image.

In terms of my theory, such dialogues are viewed as often constituting a development of the transformational process and being in keeping with the language centre's biologically evolved tendency to conceptualize and rationalize information. In this way the *causation issue*, referred to in section 2 of this introduction (what is it that motivates the use of language to explicate the visual image, etc.), is seen as being partially resolved.

8   CONCLUDING REMARKS

Perhaps the major contribution I have made to understanding the relations between the arts and cognition is to have constructed a theory of picture perception and aesthetic response primarily based upon neuropsychological data. I do not pretend, however, to have added anything 'scientific' (in the form of personally conducted experiments, for example) to neuropsychology itself. My (interdisciplinary) strategy has been, rather, to draw reasoned conclusions from the field in the hope that these can contribute to the beginnings of a relatively empirical framework capable of illuminating our relations to the arts.

When writing this book I was faced with the problem of whether to first detail the more important neuropsychological evidence and the procedural bases developed to achieve it. On the one hand, including this information could appear redundant to the reader familiar with neuropsychology; on the other, not including it would clearly prove problematic to the reader unfamiliar with the field. On reflection, it seemed to me that I had no option but to include the information given the central role it plays in my later arguments. I wish to emphasize, therefore, the necessarily expository nature of my opening chapters which pave the way for any original contributions made in subsequent chapters.

9 CHAPTER SUMMARY

In chapter 1 (The biological and procedural bases of neuropsychological research) I review the more essential aspects of the brain's biology relevant to neuropsychology and the procedures it has developed to reach its conclusions. In chapter 2 (The experimental evidence) I review the more important of these conclusions.

In chapter 3 (The possible origins of cerebral specialization) I review evidence relevant to the ontogeny and phylogeny of cerebral lateralization and draw conclusions as to why it is that the right hemisphere is particularly adept at processing spatially oriented information.

These three opening chapters enable me to hypothesize in chapter 4 (The right-hemisphere cognitive paradigm) that the right hemisphere is the biological seat of a distinct cognitive paradigm suited to directly and intuitively processing certain classes of visual-spatial information (including pictorial information) without reference to left-hemisphere associated modes of processing.

I substantiate this hypothesis in chapter 5 (Children's drawing) by arguing that we can gain insights into the nature of adult picture perception by observing the way in which children construct their drawing.

Chapter 6 (The languages of art) is concerned with three themes. The first centres around arguing against those theories of picture perception which contend that we need to learn to see pictures in something like the same way we learn a language. The second centres around arguing against those theories which contend that our proper appreciation of pictures is contingent upon forms of linguistically imparted knowledge. The third theme centres around the *translation issue* raised in section 2 of this introduction, that is, the question of the extent to which language can plausibly explicate the representational visual image.

In chapter 7 (A transformational theory of aesthetics) I hypothesize that our dominantly right-hemisphere associated perceptions of a representational image's full existential life can cause a series of compensatory/adaptive cognitions and behaviours which transform the image into appearing to generate an experience I describe as affective import. Because affective import is habitually experienced as being generated by certain works of visual art, and because it is perceived as being of a special kind, it is often associated with what has been traditionally defined as aesthetic experience. Although generally conceded to be enigmatic, the experience nonetheless prompts linguistic discourses centred around establishing its nature and the nature of its object, for my purposes, the representational visual image.

In chapter 8 (Art and aesthetic experience) I qualify my theory in terms of more traditional theories of art and aesthetics, particularly those advanced by Berleant and Bullough.

In chapter 9 (The transformational planes) I formalize my theory by dividing its processes into ten hypothetical (cognitive) stages which I term planes. These show a development which begins with our dominantly right-hemisphere and conclude with our dominantly left-hemisphere associated modes of cognitive processing.

The appendix (Psychoanalysis and art) differentiates my views from those of the paediatrician Donald Winnicott and the art critic Peter Fuller.

Chapter One

THE BIOLOGICAL AND PROCEDURAL BASES OF NEUROPSYCHOLOGY

1.1 INTRODUCTION

I have proposed that neuropsychology can illuminate certain mental competences that have a bearing on the meaning of art. This opening chapter clarifies the physical bases of the brain relevant to neuropsychology and reviews the more essential procedures it has developed to reach its findings. I shall first make a few opening remarks concerning the definition and implications of neuropsychology.

It has long been established that aspects of cognition which would be difficult to study in the healthy individual under laboratory conditions may break down in a circumscribed manner as a result of brain injury, surgery or disease. The core of neuropsychological research proceeds from a study of the clinical data provided by such cases. Even so, because neuropsychology is concerned in general with how mental life and human behaviour is related to the structure of the brain, the study of the healthy individual is not excluded from its research, as Dimond indicates.

> We are certainly not going to exclude knowledge merely because it comes from somewhere else such as the study of animals with experimental lesions of the brain or the study of the normal person who has his brain in one piece.
>
> (Dimond 1978: 4)

Taken collectively, neuropsychology's findings clearly indicate that the human brain possesses qualitatively distinct modes of cognitive processing that can be cerebrally localized. It is for this reason that it is often seen as complementing faculty psychology. In recent years, however, perhaps the most significant and certainly the most dramatic insights regarding cerebral localization of function have come from experiments conducted on commissurotomy or 'split-brain' subjects.[1] This branch of neuropsychology is termed lateralization research because of its assumption that certain higher level mental competences are lateralized to either the left or right cerebral hemispheres. Nonetheless, in keeping with the general description of neuropsychology, lateralization research includes the study of the extent to which competences are lateralized in the cerebrally intact human brain.

Cerebral lateralization of function should not be taken to mean, however, that cerebrally 'normal' individuals act out dualistically motivated lives where the left hand has no knowledge of what the right is doing, as it were. Such cases have been known to occur, but only in the commissurotomized and then only rarely.[2] As Roger Sperry, the leading investigator in the field, indicates, those who find insights gained from lateralization research should be wary, because:

> In some cases the conclusions, along with the growing wave
> of semi-popular extrapolations and speculations, concerning
> the 'left brain' versus 'right brain' functions, call for a word of
> caution ... in the normal state, the two hemispheres appear to
> work closely together as a unit.

(Sperry 1982: 1225)

Many have heeded Sperry's advice, ranging from those involved in direct experimentation in the field (Bryden 1982, for example), to those concerned with its implications for other fields (art education, for example; see Youngblood, 1979), or art in general (Schweiger 1985, for example).[3]

Nonetheless, inherent in Sperry's caution is the implication that successful cognition is contingent upon a co-operation of the hemispheres' modes of functioning. From this implication I shall argue in later chapters that when the hemispheres are presented with certain forms of pictorial information, their associated modes of processing do not necessarily work in harmony. But these are early times in this book and the purpose of this introductory chapter is not to overly speculate but to clarify the essential bases from which neuropsychology operates.

1.2 THE CEREBRAL CORTEX

Higher mental functioning in humans is associated with the cerebral cortex, a deeply fissured mantle of the brain divided into two visually like areas known as the left and right cerebral hemispheres. Each hemisphere is subdivided into four major areas known as the occipital, temporal, parietal, and frontal lobes.[4] The mirror-image nature of the cortex reflects the left-right symmetry of the body. However, although the control of basic body movement and sensation is symmetrically distributed between the hemispheres, the control mechanisms operate in reverse, as it were. In general, the left hemisphere controls the right side of the body, the right hemisphere the left, thereby conceptually establishing a cross-fashion or 'X' functional mode. This is physically substantiated by the fact that the left hemisphere's neural connections receive and generate signals primarily to the right side of the body and vice versa.

As a result of this X functional mode, if inputted information is confined to one side of the body it is initially primarily *contralaterally* registered by the cortex. For example, tactile information experienced by the right hand is primarily registered by the left hemisphere, whereas information from the left hand is registered by the right hemisphere. The notable exception is olfactory information which is *ipsilaterally* registered. That is, the left nostril transmits information to the left hemisphere, the right nostril transmits information to the right hemisphere.

The same X functional mode applies to the generation of basic body movement, that is, the brain's basic capacity to control motor skills. Motor skills for the movement in the hand or foot, for example, primarily emanate from the hemisphere located on the opposite side of the body. The exception is the movement of facial muscles which are controlled by both hemispheres.

It should be emphasized, however, that the way in which the brain controls basic body movement and sensation should not be confused with the way in which it processes and subsequently responds to higher order information, in which case it displays a marked *asymmetry of function*. In right-handers, for example, it is almost exclusively the case that the hemisphere controlling the dominant hand is also the one controlling speech, that is, the left hemisphere. There is, however, a great deal of accumulated evidence which argues that, in the case of the right-hander drawing a picture, for example, the guiding spatially oriented knowledge

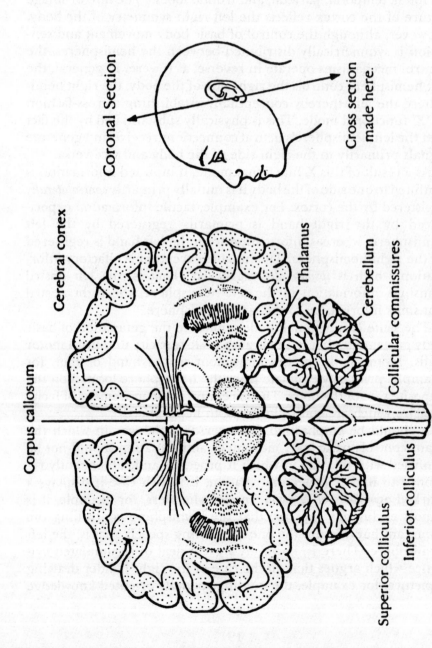

Figure 1 Extent of the separation of the brain following forebrain commissurotomy

Source: Sperry 1964b. Copyright 1964 Scientific American Inc.

emanates from the right hemisphere.

From this it follows as a general rule that the hemisphere which generates the basic body movement relevant to a particular task is not necessarily the one most capable of its cognition.

At this point, however, Sperry's indication that the hemispheres normally function as a unit should be emphasized. This is because they are linked to the spinal column and peripheral nerves through a common brain stem and because, above all, they are linked by the corpus callosum, a large band of nerve fibres embedded between the hemispheres. These connections are collectively known as the commissures. Most of the evidence indicates, however, that it is primarily the corpus callosum that enables higher order information to pass in some form between the hemispheres. As a result, even if information is initially exclusively registered and processed by one hemisphere, it can be transferred to its partner hemisphere (exactly what transformational laws this transference might involve is still unknown).

The exception is found in the commissurotomized because, with the corpus callosum disconnected, information can no longer be directly exchanged between the hemispheres (Figure 1). This disconnection means that the hemispheres become functionally isolated from each other thereby enabling their respective cognitive characteristics to be individually studied.[5] This study requires complex procedures to ensure that information inputted to the cortex is registered exclusively by the hemisphere under investigation, that is, the information must be *unilaterally* registered.

At this point, then, something should be said about the procedures developed by neuropsychology to confine information to one hemisphere. Some of the procedures used to study the brain-damaged are also used to study the normal subject.

1.3 TACHISTOSCOPIC PRESENTATION

The unilateral registration of visual information presents the researcher with a particularly complex problem. This is because in both the normal and brain-damaged subject each retina can relay information to the cortex so that it is both *contralaterally* and *ipsilaterally* registered.[6] That is, the left half of each retina, which scans the right half of the visual field, sends impulses to the left hemisphere; impulses from the left half of the visual field are transmitted by the right half of each retina to the right hemisphere. What this amounts to for experimental purposes is that if the subject fixates on a central point in front, the right hemisphere exclusively registers information presented to the left visual field (LVF) whereas the left hemisphere exclusively registers information presented to the right visual field (RVF). However, to ensure correct hemispherical registration the speed at which information is presented to either visual field has to be faster than the saccadic eye movements of the subject. This is because if their focus strays even momentarily from the central point to either visual field, the information will be *bilaterally* registered, that is, registered by both hemispheres.

The need to present visual information at speed necessitated the development of the tachistoscope, a device which flashes information to either side of a screen with a marked central point. In this way, when focusing on this point, information flashed to either side falls exclusively within the subject's respective visual fields and is therefore unilaterally registered as required (Figure 2).

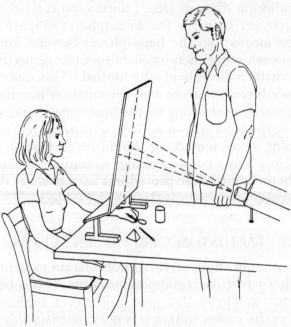

Figure 2 The basic testing arrangement used to lateralize visual and tactile information and allow tactile responses

Source: Springer and Deutsch 1981.

While tachistoscopic presentation to the commissurotomized solved the problem of limiting information to either hemisphere, the speed at which it had to be presented limited experimentation; that is, the subject could not be expected to detail a response to information viewed for only a split second. This limitation was overcome, however, when Zaidel (1975) developed a new method of restricting visual information to one hemisphere. It utilizes a device described as the Z contact lens occluder (the Z lens) which permits subjects to freely move their eyes when examining information and at the same time ensures that it is registered by only one hemisphere.

The Z lens therefore makes it possible to view information for as long as necessary to an experiment yet also allows it to be exclusively registered by the hemisphere under investigation. The use of the Z lens has led to some of the most important lateralization research studies centred on establishing the right hemisphere's level of consciousness, as we shall see in the next chapter.

1.4 CROSS-MODAL REFERENCING[7]

Early tachistoscopic presentation involving commissurotomy subjects quickly established that information flashed to the LVF (right-hemisphere registered) went verbally unacknowledged. This was predictable because it was known that, although the right hemisphere possesses some capacity to understand language, in the majority of cases the speech centres are left-hemisphere located. Researchers therefore had to find extra-verbal methods of eliciting from the subject the extent to which information had been registered and comprehended by the right hemisphere.

One of the commonest methods was to flash an image of a well-known item – a spoon, for example – and then to ask the subject to select, using the left hand, a real spoon from an array of items hidden from view.[8] In most instances, the subject correctly identified the item by feeling its shape and contours (Figure 2). This clearly indicated that, although the item's image had gone verbally unacknowledged, it had, in fact, been right-hemisphere registered and comprehended. Nonetheless, unless the item was shown to the left speech hemisphere, it continued to remain verbally unacknowledged by the right.

Other methods of eliciting the extent to which tachistoscopically presented information had been right-hemisphere registered and comprehended were developed by researchers, leading to some intriguing results.

1.5 CROSS-CUING

As lateralization research developed, certain inconsistencies in the findings began to occur with increasing frequency. Subjects initially unable to verbally identify items hidden from view but held in the left hand began to name some items. Interpretations of these results ranged from the suggestion that over time the right hemisphere had developed a speech capacity to the suggestion that information was being transmitted between the hemispheres via the lesser communication pathways such as the lower brain stem.

Gazzaniga and Hillyard (1971) offered a simpler explanation for the inconsistency which they termed cross-cuing. This refers to the commissurotomy subject's attempt to use all the available clues to make information available to both hemispheres. For example, it was found that if the left hand selected a comb or a toothbrush, the subject would often stroke the brush or comb. Because the ensuing sound became readily available to the left speech hemisphere, this often enabled the item to be verbally identified. Taking into account such instances, it was proposed as a general rule that when the channels which normally allow direct interhemispheric communication are disconnected by surgery, cross-cuing provides a method for one hemisphere to communicate to its partner hemisphere what it is experiencing by indirect means. It was also proposed that the tendency to cross-cue offers an explanation for why it is that, in everyday activity, the commissurotomized appear relatively unaffected by their radical surgery.

1.6 DICHOTIC LISTENING

Techniques to lateralize distinct classes of auditory information have also been used to study hemispheric differences both in the normal and brain-damaged subject. As with vision, however, the unilateral registration of auditory information for experimental purposes presents the researcher with a complex problem. This is because the auditory pathways from each ear reach the hemispheres from both contralateral and ipsilateral routes. From this it follows that, in both the normal and brain-damaged subject, information should be registered by both hemispheres regardless of which ear initially receives it.[9]

In contradiction to this, however, Kimura (1961a, 1961b) noticed that under certain conditions subjects were more accurate at identifying words presented to the right ear than they were at identifying ones presented to the left. Kimura was using the dichotic listening procedure in which subjects listen to two distinct auditory messages simultaneously inputted to each ear. Her experiment was designed to compare the performances of left and right temporal lobe damaged subjects and normal subjects.

The auditory stimuli used by Kimura consisted of pairs of spoken digits, 'one' and 'nine', for example.[10] The members of each pair were aligned for simultaneity of onset and were recorded on separate channels of sound tape. Subjects listened through stereo headphones to trials consisting of three pairs of digits presented in rapid succession. After each trial they were asked to recall as many of the six previously presented digits as possible in any order.

Results indicated that subjects with left temporal lobe damage performed worse than those with damage to the right lobe. Regardless of where the damage was located, however, subjects typically reported digits presented to the right ear more accurately than those presented to the left. The right ear advantage was also found to exist in the normal, control subjects.

The observation that subjects with left temporal lobe damage performed worse than those with damage to the right was predictable. Kimura's initial dichotic listening presentations involved the capacity to understand and produce speech, which, as we have seen, are dominantly left-hemisphere functions. It followed, therefore, that speech comprehension and production were more likely to have been disrupted in subjects with left-hemisphere damage. The observation that the ears performed asymmetrically, however, proved surprising to Kimura because she was aware that the auditory pathways from each ear have direct access to both hemispheres. Therefore, even if speech could only be processed by the left hemisphere, the left ear should have performed equally as well as the right; that is, left-ear inputted information should have had equal access to the left hemisphere via the ipsilateral route and it should therefore have been recalled as successfully as

right-ear inputted information. Kimura's subsequent explanation
for this inconsistency led to the construction of a model of ear asymmetry that has remained viable to the present.

Kimura noted from animal studies that the contralateral projections from ear to brain are stronger than the ipsilateral projections
(Rosenweig 1951). From this evidence she proposed that when two
distinct auditory stimuli are simultaneously inputted to each ear

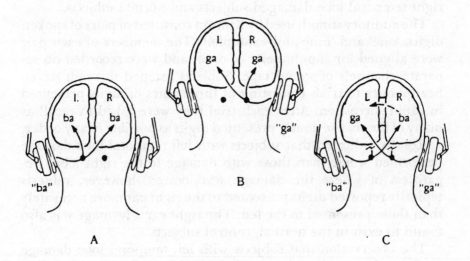

Figure 3 Kimura's model of dichotic listening in normal subjects. A. Monaural presentation to the left ear is sent to the right hemisphere by way
of contralateral pathways and to the left hemisphere by way of ipsilateral
pathways. The subject reports the syllable 'ba' accurately. B. Monaural
presentation to the right ear is sent to the left hemisphere by way of contralateral pathways and to the right hemisphere by way of ipsilateral pathways. The subject reports the syllable 'ga' accurately. C. In dichotic
presentation, ipsilateral pathways are suppressed, so 'ga' goes only to the
left (speech) hemisphere and 'ba' to the right hemisphere. The syllable
'ba' is accessible to the left (speech) hemisphere only through the commissures. As a consequence, 'ga' is usually reported more accurately than 'ba'
(a right-ear advantage).

Source: Springer and Deutsch 1981

the strength of the signal to the contralateral pathway is exaggerated and suppresses or occludes the signal relayed via the ipsilateral route. In experimental conditions, therefore, when stimuli is simultaneously presented to both ears it is primarily contralaterally registered in keeping with the X functional mode. Given this assumption, it was subsequently possible for Kimura to explain her initial findings that subjects were more accurate at identifying words or digits presented to the right ear.

Her explanation went as follows: under dichotic presentation conditions the stimulus inputted to the left ear can theoretically reach the left (language) hemisphere in one of two ways – either via the ipsilateral route or via the contralateral pathways to the right hemisphere and then across to the left hemisphere via the corpus callosum. The stimulus inputted to the right ear, however, has a less circuitous path to follow before it reaches the left hemisphere because it gains direct access along the contralateral route. Since the contralateral signal is stronger, the stimulus arrives at the left hemisphere for processing with a clear advantage over the left-ear inputted stimulus which arrives by the longer route in the way described. Kimura reasoned that from this a left-hemisphere advantage for words emerges (Figure 3).

Kimura's early dichotic listening experiments were designed to test the brain's capacity to process linguistically oriented information. As we shall see presently, subsequent experiments clearly indicate a left ear and therefore primarily right-hemisphere registered and processing advantage for classes of nonverbal or paralinguistic auditory information. This indicates that ear asymmetry relates to the nature of the information presented thereby substantiating the view that the hemispheres possess qualitatively different modes of cognitive processing.

1.7   LATERAL EYE MOVEMENT STUDIES

In the course of his practice as a clinical psychologist, Day observed that patients consistently looked either to the left or right when answering questions. From this observation he hypothesized that the direction of lateral eye movements (LEM) could be associated with certain personality characteristics (Day 1964). Several years on, Bakan published a paper supporting this hypothesis and added that eye movements could be related to hemispheric asymmetry of function (Bakan 1969). This new hypothesis was based on the knowledge that eye movements to either the left or right are motor-controlled by the centres in the frontal lobe of the contralateral hemisphere. From this it was reasoned that cognitions occurring dominantly in one hemisphere would activate eye movements to the opposite side of the face in the proven X functional mode. It followed, therefore, that eye movements could be seen as an index of the relative activities of the hemispheres in the individual. Subjects who typically look to the left are those for whom the right hemisphere dominates, whereas those who look to the right are those for whom the left dominates.

Bakan thought of the direction of lateral eye movements as a stable characteristic of an individual. Later researchers exploring lateral eye movements as an index of hemispheric activity considered the role played by the type of question used to elicit a response. It was reasoned that questions requiring an analysis of words and their meaning would engage the left hemisphere, whereas questions involving spatial relations or musical skills would engage the right hemisphere. In the former case the subject would look to the left, in the latter to the right. Results of lateral eye movement studies are reviewed in the next chapter.

Lateral eye movement studies appealed to lateralization researchers because the approach indicated the possibility of investigating left and right hemisphere competences without using the standard tachistoscopic presentation or dichotic listening procedures. However, a significant review of the field has argued that the link between hemispheric activity and eye movement is indirect and tenuous (Ehrlichman and Weinberger 1979). The critics are sceptical regarding what constitutes a 'left-hemisphere' as distinct from a 'right-hemisphere' question; that is, they argue if it is necessary to define left- or right-hemisphere activity in terms of the questions that produce the expected results, the logical problem of establishing a relation between eye movement and brain asymmetry is essentially circular in nature.

The remaining most relevant procedures developed to study cerebral asymmetry of function are: electrophysiological measures, studies of regional blood flow and the Wada test. These have been of value in physiologically substantiating some of the psychological insights gained from the non-invasive procedures reviewed.

1.8   ELECTROPHYSIOLOGICAL MEASURES OF CEREBRAL ASYMMETRY

In 1929 the Austrian psychiatrist Hans Burger discovered that patterns of electrical activity in the brain could be recorded by electrodes placed at various locations on the human scalp. These patterns are called electroencephalogram (EEG), literally meaning 'electrical brain wiring'. Burger was able to demonstrate that EEG recordings originate in the brain itself and are not merely due to scalp musculature response. EEG recordings were typically made from electrodes placed at different locations along the top or to one side only of the head. This was because it was generally assumed that the brain's electrical activity would be identical on both sides. Devices to record EEG were increasingly used in clinical situations as researchers demonstrated that brain abnormalities such as epilepsy and tumours are accompanied by distinctive patterns of electrical activity.

Studies on the first commissurotomy patients, operated on in the 1960s, clearly indicated the functional asymmetry of the respective hemispheres. Taking this into account, Galin and Ornstein applied EEG techniques to study brain asymmetry in the normal subject and relate it to the task being performed (1972). Their reasoning was that, although lateralization research had shown the verbal and spatial cognitive systems function independently, few studies existed that attempted to evaluate their degrees of interaction in the normal subject. Galin and Ornstein's prediction was that, in most ordinary activities, rather than integrating distinct cognitive modes, we simply alternate between them. In a subject performing a verbal or spatial task, therefore, one hemisphere or the other would dominate.[11]

EEG signals were recorded from the respective hemispheres while college students were engaged in either linguistically or spatially oriented tasks. When subjects engaged in linguistic tasks, alpha rhythms were reduced in the left hemisphere but remained strong in the right, whereas an opposite effect was recorded when subjects engaged in spatial tasks. Because alpha rhythms are not associated with concentrated brain activity it was concluded that the hemisphere with the strongest alpha rhythm was the less active in relation to a task.[12] All of the subjects showed a change in EEG activity in the predicted direction. Galin and Ornstein were therefore successful in showing a link between brain activity and the type of task performed thereby adding to the evidence that the hemispheres possess qualitatively distinct modes of cognitive processing.

Because EEG is an overall, continuous measure of brain activity, however, difficulties initially arose in observing subtle changes in the EEG relative to specific tasks. This was because the changes were often obscured by the 'noise' of the brain's general activity. Since early EEG recording, the problem of differentiating genuine EEG responses from general brain noise has been largely overcome with the use of computers which average waveform recordings following repeated presentations of the same task; that is, random noise is negated by the averaging process while the electrical activity relevant to the task remains consistent and emerges as what is known as the evoked potential (EP). Results are reviewed in the next chapter.

1.9   BLOOD FLOW IN THE HEMISPHERES

The measurement of blood flow in the hemispheres has also been used to measure cerebral activity and localization of function. Cognitive changes in different regions of the brain appear to relate to the amount of blood flowing through these regions. This has made it possible to identify and study the cognitive interaction of various brain regions by measuring their blood flow.

Modern techniques of measuring blood flow in the conscious subject were developed by Lassan and Ingvar (1972) who injected a special radioactive isotope (xenon 133) into the blood stream and subsequently monitored the blood flow with a battery of detectors arranged near the surface of the head. The technique, originally used with patients requiring the test for medical purposes, has been refined to the point where subjects can breath a special air-xenon mixture and have their blood flow monitored by special detectors.

Current work on cerebral blood flow indicates that complex tasks typically involve increased patterns of activation in several areas of each hemisphere. It should be noted, however, that techniques are insufficiently accurate to provide detailed information about the activities of the deepest areas of the brain. The xenon 133 method is just one of several methods used for brain-scanning.

1.10   THE WADA TEST

In the Wada test a small tube is inserted into the cartoid artery on one side of the patient's neck thereby allowing sodium amytal to be injected into the artery. The drug is used to temporarily anaesthetize one hemisphere at a time and is typically used to determine which hemisphere controls speech in patients about to undergo brain surgery (Wada and Rasmussen 1960). This method has also provided important information concerning the relationship of handedness to hemispheric asymmetry and the effects of early brain damage (Rasmussen and Milner 1977).

Chapter Two

THE EXPERIMENTAL EVIDENCE

2.1 INTRODUCTION

My opening chapter was primarily concerned with reviewing the biological and procedural bases of neuropsychological research; in this chapter I review the experimental evidence itself. However, since interest in the biological basis of mental life increased dramatically following the split-brain operations of the 1960s, it is clearly impossible to detail every aspect of the field, or for that matter, to detail every study reviewed here. I have, therefore, selected only those studies which, in my view, encapsulate the nature and implications of neuropsychology, and detailed only those pertinent to illustrating my later conclusions.

Whenever possible, I have classified the data in accordance with those procedures employed to achieve it, tachistoscopic presentation as distinct from dichotic listening, for example, although some overlap is bound to occur. This is because the procedures, although distinct, typically obtain their results by involving several of the subject's sense modalities. For instance, while the stimulus involved in tachistoscopic presentation is necessarily visual it is often accompanied by audition in the form of the examiner's oral questioning, whereas the subject's response can include the use of touch, manipulospatial abilities in general, and speech.[1] From this it follows that the results from tachistoscopic presentation share aspects in common with those obtained from other examining techniques involving subjects' like sense modalities, and by implication, mental faculties.

2.2 THE BEGINNINGS OF LATERALIZATION RESEARCH

Over a century ago, Broca (1861) dispelled the widely held notion that the human brain was bilateral by presenting clinical data indicating that the speech faculty is typically confined to the left hemisphere.[2] Subsequent research by Wernicke indicated that the left hemisphere also plays a central role in speech comprehension, reading, and writing. Although Jackson (1874) speculated that the right hemisphere plays an important role in visual ideation and emotion, for the following hundred years, with few exceptions, research concentrated on exploring the role played in cognition by the left hemisphere because of its association with language functions.[3]

In 1956, Myers reported results from a series of animal experiments (Myers 1956; Sperry 1959). The research had involved sectioning either a cat's optic chiasm or both the chiasm and corpus callosum. In the former case the prediction was that, although the sectioned chiasm would allow information to be unilaterally registered, the information could transfer to the partner hemisphere via the (intact) corpus callosum. In the latter case the prediction was that the unilaterally registered information would remain lateralized because, with the corpus callosum disconnected, no transfer of information to the partner hemisphere should be possible. Results confirmed expectations. Further, with the corpus callosum disconnected it was found that the respective hemispheres could be taught different and sometimes conflicting discriminations. This result indicated that the corpus callosum was the animals' major inter-hemispheric communication pathway and that the respective hemispheres were capable of independent function.

The emergence of Bogen and Vogel's complete commissurotomy patients (Bogen and Vogel 1962; Fisher et al. 1965) provided Sperry and Gazzaniga with suitable human subjects to test some of the hypotheses that had resulted from the incipient animal research experiments (Gazzaniga 1970; Gazzaniga and LeDoux 1978). Their investigations sparked renewed interest in cerebral asymmetry of function and led to a reappraisal of the role played in cognition by the right 'mute' hemisphere.

2.3 EARLY RESULTS OF TACHISTOSCOPIC PRESENTATION

Until the implications of Sperry and Gazzaniga's incipient research were fully realized, the classic view of left hemisphere cerebral dominance was still widely held. Because the accumulated data from Broca's research onwards indicated that the right hemisphere lacked speech, it had been assumed by extrapolation that it was also word deaf and blind and typically incapable of symbol-processing in general. Even as the clinical data increasingly suggested that the right hemisphere possessed not only an ability to comprehend language but also its own specialized abilities, these were ascribed to its sensory and motor executive realms.

Early indications of the right-hemisphere specialities in the lateral lesion data, such as facial recognition, dressing, making block designs, drawing three-dimensional cubes, and so forth, had been ascribed to asymmetry primarily in the sensory and motor executive realms rather than in higher cognitive levels. These right hemispheric functions were referred to as 'visuospatial', 'constructional', or 'praxic'.

(Sperry 1982: 1224)

As the clinical data accumulated, however, Sperry became convinced that the right hemisphere was, in fact, capable of functioning independently and that it exhibited signs of consciousness (Sperry 1964a, 1964b, 1966, 1968). His conviction was essentially based on the observation that, when verbally questioned, the left hemisphere remained incognizant of the higher level mental performances ascribed to the right hemisphere in the experimental situation.[4] By 1968 we find Sperry concluding:

In the split-brain syndrome we deal with two separate spheres of conscious awareness, i.e. two separate conscious entities or minds running in parallel in the same cranium, each with its own sensations, perceptions, cognitive processes, learning experiences, memories, and so on.

(Sperry 1968: 318)

This conclusion that the mechanisms of consciousness may be doubly represented following brain bisection did not go unchallenged and still remains a contentious issue. Early on, Eccles (1965) asserted that the psychological capabilities of the right hemisphere were best described as 'automatisms', a view from which he has not radically departed (Eccles 1980). MacKay (1972) argued unless it could be shown that each isolated hemisphere had its own independent systems for subjectively assigning values to events and setting goals and response properties, the split brain could not be thought of as a split mind. Significantly, when one considers his early collaboration with Sperry, Gazzaniga subsequently voiced similar reservations concerning the right hemisphere's level of consciousness, as we shall see in later chapters in some detail.[5]

In 1970 Gazzaniga published a detailed account of his early research on the split-brain syndrome.[6] The clinical data in the account (74–126) resulted from tests conducted on three of Bogen and Vogel's complete commissurotomy patients. The tests, centred around tachistoscopic presentation, were designed to establish the right hemisphere's ability to write, visually comprehend stimuli, comprehend nouns, adjectives, and verb structures, comprehend spoken words and execute spelling, and to calculate. In conclusion, Gazzaniga noted, 'Information perceived exclusively or generated exclusively by the minor (right) hemisphere could be communicated neither in speech nor in writing' (125).

The results nonetheless indicated to Gazzaniga that the right hemisphere possessed some linguistic ability, 'In contrast to the highly lateralized organization of verbal expression, the comprehension of language, both spoken and written, was found to be represented in the minor hemisphere as well as in the major hemisphere' (125). We are also informed that the right hemisphere performed well in tasks involving word and object association, sorting, retrieval, and exhibited other higher order mental capacities. However, Gazzaniga is mystified as to the right hemisphere's true function:

> The cerebral taxonomy of life is of enormous interest but still leaves unanswered ... what the predominant function is of one entire half of the human cerebrum. The meagre list of its assets unearthed to date hardly appears inadequate to explain its role in the light of the amount of neural tissue involved.
>
> (Gazzaniga 1970: 142)

In an attempt to qualify the apparent meagreness of the right hemisphere's assets, Gazzaniga speculates that it could function to allow initially left-hemisphere processed verbal information the necessary 'processing space' or 'reverberation time' thereby, 'enabling the system to check and cross-check the proposition and subsequently possibly to initiate qualifying remarks' (143). Consistent with this view, continues Gazzaniga, is the suggestion by MacKay that the right hemisphere might serve to qualify left-hemisphere produced statements, 'The idea here is that the right hemisphere would be "thinking" of the qualifications of the ongoing statements by listening to the left hemisphere and then serving notice on the left hemisphere when to qualify or modify the content of a particular declaration' (142). It is pointed out that this essentially pragmatically oriented view of right-hemisphere language function is supported by Hall *et al.* (1968) who reported that patients with right-hemisphere cerebral lesions did not qualify statements to the extent observed in those with lesions to the left hemisphere.

Subsequent clinical data generally supports the case that the right hemisphere plays a pragmatic (and semantic) role in speech production. Deglin (1976) observed that patients with right-hemisphere damage, while capable of making mathematical sense, often became garrulous as if their sentences lacked meaning; intonation became less expressive and often acquired a nasal twang or became utterly unnatural. In a more general vein, Jakobson's review of the brain's relation to language (1980) indicates that the right hemisphere plays a central role in processing paralinguistic phenomena, as we shall see further on in this chapter.

2.4   THE RIGHT HEMISPHERE'S CONTRIBUTION TO COGNITION

Results of early experiments designed to elicit the nature of right hemisphere function which did not concentrate on its linguistic abilities indicated that it specializes in processing spatially oriented information. Hecaen and Angelergues (1962) concluded that right-hemisphere strokes make facial recognition (proposagnosia) difficult. Kimura (1963) concluded that right-hemisphere damage affects the capacity for maze learning and the recognition of nonsense figures. Bogen (1969a) reported a series of drawings produced by some of his commissurotomy patients who had been asked to copy relatively simple objects using each hand in turn.

The drawings clearly exhibit a left-hand and, because of the X functional mode, right-hemisphere advantage for this activity.[7]

Hecaen and Sauguet (1971) conducted a series of tests on right- and left-handed brain-lesioned subjects. The results overwhelmingly indicate a right-hemisphere advantage in the right-handed for spatially oriented tasks. They are particularly significant when it is taken into account that 560 subjects were involved in the tests.[8]

Nebes (1972) found that the right hemisphere of commissurotomy subjects was significantly superior to the left in tasks designed to measure the capacity to synthetically process spatially involved information. Subjects were required to manually examine three geometric designs, out of view, while looking at a visually fragmented sketch of one of the designs. The task was to determine which of the three manually examined designs matched the visually fragmented sketch. The right hand (left hemisphere) performed the task at no more than chance level (33 per cent), while the left hand (right hemisphere) scores ranged between 75 per cent and 90 per cent correct. This result clearly indicates a right-hemisphere advantage in processing spatially oriented information synthetically.

In a later study conducted by Nebes (1973) the separated hemispheres were required to judge whether arrays of dots appeared to form vertical or horizontal lines. The right hemisphere was found to be superior to the left in this task, from which it was concluded that the right hemisphere specializes in Gestalt perception.

As experimental techniques developed, chimeric-figure studies were used to understand right-hemisphere function. In a significant study, Levy *et al.* (1972) constructed three chimeric faces of young men. (A chimeric face is constructed from two half image faces, left or right, of different people.) The faces were tachistoscopically presented to the (commissurotomy) subjects' respective visual fields thereby ensuring the unilateral registration of only one half of the whole face. The subjects were subsequently asked to point, using either hand, to a face from a choice array displayed in free vision which resembled the tachistoscopically presented chimeric face. The array consisted of normal faces from which any one half had been combined to form the chimeric face stimuli. Regardless of the hand used to point, the subjects overwhelmingly selected the face that had been right-hemisphere registered in the tachistoscopic presentation.[9]

These results indicated that the right hemisphere was superior to the left in recognizing faces, thereby substantiating the earlier results reported by Hecaen and Angelergues regarding proposagnosia. However, in the Levy study, when the left hemisphere was forced to play a role in the task, that is, when a *verbal* response was demanded, it named the half of the chimeric face presented to the RVF and therefore left-hemisphere registered.

In a further test in the series the researchers presented chimeric stimuli formed by dividing and subsequently re-combining mundane imagery (a rose, an eye, a bee, for example). The forms were tachistoscopically presented to the subjects in the way described. When pointing, they again matched the image registered by the right hemisphere but when asked to verbally identify what they had seen the majority of responses were to the left-hemisphere registered image.

From these and other chimeric studies, Levy developed the important hypothesis of cerebral *dominance* and *capacity*. Dominance refers to the tendency for one hemisphere to process information and control response, whereas capacity refers merely to the ability of a hemisphere to perform a task when required (Levy 1974; Perecman 1983: 15). In the chimeric face study reviewed here, therefore, the left hemisphere exhibited the capacity to recognize faces when a verbal acknowledgement was required but it was not dominant in this task because the overwhelming majority of responses came from the right hemisphere in the free response situation.

The use of composite faces has been used to research whether the expression of emotion is cerebrally lateralized in the normal individual. Campbell (1978) asked subjects to pose for full frontal face photographs that were subsequently divided down the midline, reversed, and re-combined to produce left and right composites of the original image. Subjects judged that the left half composite face was more 'emotional' than the right.[10]

Other studies using facial imagery have been used to understand cerebral asymmetry of emotion and expression. Borod and Caron (1980) videotaped posed facial expressions and found that subjects judged the left half as being the most expressive. Moscovitch and Olds (1982) also found that the left side of the face was more expressive than the right when communicating in both the laboratory and field setting. (For further studies concerned with the role the face plays in emotion and the nature of cerebral asymmetry of emo-

38

tion generally, see Gardner 1975; Geschwind 1976; Ley and Bryden 1979; Ross and Mesulam 1979; Cicone *et al.* 1980; Bryden 1982; Bryden and Ley 1983; Borod *et al.* 1983.)

2.5 TWO SEMINAL EXPERIMENTS INVOLVING TACHISTOSCOPIC PRESENTATION

Before reviewing evidence relevant to the lateralization of auditory phenomena, two seminal experiments involving tachistoscopic presentation are worth detailing. The first comes from the series conducted by Gazzaniga and LeDoux (1978) on Wilson's commissurotomy patients; the second from the series conducted by Sperry *et al.* (1979) on two of Vogel's original commissurotomy patients.

In 1970, Donald Wilson performed a new series of commissurotomy operations. In the first phase of the series, Wilson invariably sectioned the entire corpus callosum and anterior commissure; in the second phase, only the corpus callosum. Wilson's patients, who were subsequently tested for cerebral lateralization by Gazzaniga and LeDoux, thus provided neuropsychology with a unique research opportunity. (See LeDoux *et al.* 1977a, 1977b, and Risse *et al.* 1977.)

The test most widely reported involved the subject P.S. who had sustained complete sectioning of the corpus callosum with the anterior commissure left intact. P.S. was of particular interest to the researchers because extended testing indicated that his right hemisphere, although typically incapable of speech, exhibited an above average language capacity relative to other subjects who had sustained similar surgery.

The test conducted on P.S. that I shall review here is significant for several reasons. First, as in the Levy chimeric-figure studies, it involved simultaneous tachistoscopic presentation of visual stimuli to the respective hemispheres. In advance of the Levy studies, however, correct right-hemisphere response to the stimuli clearly involved the activation of sophisticated mental operations including cross-modal associations, long term memory, and so forth. In other words, successful response to the stimuli required higher level forms of cognition typically associated with consciousness. Second, because of the (tachistoscopically) divided nature of the stimuli, results indicated that P.S.'s left hemisphere, in virtue of its speech capacity, was capable of vicariously subsuming his right-

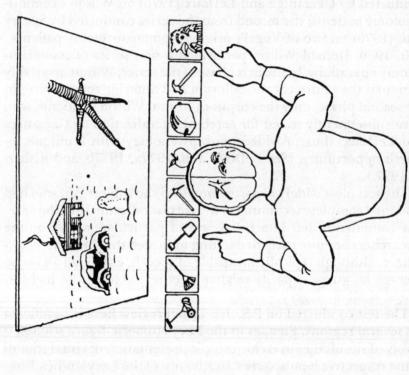

Figure 4 The method used in presenting two different cognitive tasks simultaneously, one to each hemisphere

Source: Gazzaniga and LeDoux 1978

hemisphere response. Third, results from this and other tests conducted on P.S. led the researchers to formulate a radically new
theory of behaviour and memory (later developed by Gazzaniga
1985) both of which, it is argued, have significant implications for
the cerebrally intact or 'normal' individual.

P.S. was tested with pairs of pictures simultaneously tachistoscopically presented to his respective visual fields thereby ensuring
unilateral hemispheric registration. Immediately following the
presentation, he was required to point to those pictures presented
in a choice array that in some way matched the tachistoscopically
presented pictures. For example, an image of a house and car surrounded by snow could well relate to a shovel image given the
practical relations between shovels and clearing snow.

In response to these (divided) presentations, P.S.'s right hand
typically chose a picture from the choice array relevant to his left-
hemisphere registered information whereas his left hand chose one
relevant to right-hemisphere registered information. This response conformed to the X functional mode and was therefore
predictable (Figure 4). Of more interest to the researchers was the
way in which P.S. verbally interpreted his dualistic responses.

> When a snow scene was presented to the right hemisphere
> and a chicken claw was presented to the left, P.S. quickly and
> dutifully responded correctly by choosing a picture of a
> chicken from a series of four cards with his right hand and a
> picture of a shovel from a series of four cards with his left
> hand. The subject was then asked, 'What did you see?' 'I saw
> a claw and I picked the chicken and you have to clean out
> the chicken shed with a shovel.'
> (Gazzaniga and LeDoux 1978: 148)

In repeated trials, similar confabulatory left-hemisphere generated responses were observed. Therefore, the left (speech)
hemisphere could accurately verbally state why it had made its
choice and would subsequently incorporate the right-hemisphere
choice (of which it knew nothing) into its 'rationalizing' verbal
framework. The researchers did of course clearly know why the
right hemisphere had made its choice – the connection between
snow clearing and shovels, for example – not *imagined* chicken sheds
and shovels. And here it should be emphasized that the left hemisphere's confabulation was verbally presented as a *statement of fact*.

Importantly, from these and other observations of P.S.'s behaviour, Gazzaniga and LeDoux go on to argue that similar verbally constructed confabulatory responses could be universal and not merely confined to the split-brain syndrome:

> We feel that the conscious verbal self is not always privy to the origins of our actions, and when it observes the person behaving for unknown reasons it attributes cause to the action as if it knows but it in fact does not. It is as if the verbal self looks out and sees what the person is doing, and from that knowledge interprets a reality.
>
> (Gazzaniga and LeDoux 1978: 149–50)

It is hypothesized further that the (left-hemisphere) verbal self's capacity to dominate all other behaviours could under certain circumstances lead to cognitive conflict, in which regard Festinger's theory of cognitive dissonance is referred to (Festinger 1957). The theory argues that when a person's beliefs, options, or attitudes are met with disagreement as a result of freely observed behaviour, a state of dissonance obtains. Therefore, if someone's verbal expressions (what they say) conflict with the way in which they behave (what they do) a cognitive schism is experienced. These schismatic states can be overcome, however, by the reorganization of personal value systems, in which case a state of consonance once more obtains.

Regarding the general implication that individuals can produce linguistically non-introspectible behaviour, Gazzaniga and Le-Doux construct a novel theory of memory. Because this theory goes some way to biologically substantiating my account of picture perception I return to it in a later chapter. For the present it is sufficient to note that, although Gazzaniga and LeDoux argue that left-hemisphere generated verbal dominance can lead to mental conflict, they nonetheless subscribe to the classic view of cerebral dominance.

> The mind is not a psychological entity but a sociological entity composed of many submental systems. What can be done surgically and through hemisphere anaesthetization are only exaggerated instances of a more general phenomenon. The uniqueness of man, in this regard, is his ability to verbalize and, in so doing, create a personal sense of conscious reality out of the multiple mental systems present.
>
> (Gazzaniga and LeDoux 1978: 151)

In other words, linguistic sophistication is viewed as being the major force in determining consciousness in the hemispheres. Therefore, because in tests other than the ones reviewed here (142–8, for example) P.S. appeared to exhibit an above average right-hemisphere language capacity, it was concluded that it *atypically* possessed consciousness:

> Because P.S. is the first split-brain patient to clearly possess double consciousness, it seems that if we could identify the factor that distinguishes his right hemisphere from the right hemisphere of other split-brain patients, we would have a major clue to the underlying nature of conscious processes. That factor is undoubtedly the extensive linguistic representation in P.S.'s right hemisphere.
>
> (Gazzaniga and LeDoux 1978: 145)[11]

Gazzaniga and LeDoux's implication that in the majority of split-brain patients the right hemisphere lacks consciousness was almost immediately questioned by results from a series of tests conducted by Sperry *et al.* (1979) using the recently developed Z lens.

As was the case with the Gazzaniga and LeDoux tests, those conducted by Sperry *et al.* were primarily designed to establish the level of consciousness in the disconnected right hemisphere. The subjects (N.G. and L.B.) were two of Vogel's complete forebrain commissurotomy patients from the 1960s (Bogen and Vogel 1962, 1963; Sperry 1968; Gazzaniga 1970). They were selected because both had suffered relatively less damage to extra commissural systems than other patients and because each had been fitted for previous studies with the Z lens. Both were right-handed and neither was known for an above average right hemisphere language capacity.

The testing procedure involved the presentation of a choice array of four to nine items consisting of pictures, line drawings, printed or written material, or photographs arranged on a card for visual inspection. In all cases the subject's vision was confined by the Z lens to the desired visual field thereby ensuring the unilateral registration of the stimuli for as long as necessary to a test. Key pictures, for which the subject may have some familiarity preference or emotional response, were inserted irregularly among neutral items. Introduction to each choice array was accompanied by leading remarks and questions from the examiner, these often being oriented so as to establish the desired mental sets and associations that would contextualize particular items on the choice card. It was assumed that both hemispheres heard and understood the examiner's verbal instructions and remarks but that only the right hemisphere had the necessary visually registered information for an appropriate response.

Following the presentation of the items, the subject was required to point to one or more in the choice array that he might recognize, most like or dislike, or might select for a given situation or reason. The subject was often asked to evaluate initial feelings about certain items by using a 'thumbs-up' or 'thumbs-down' gesture. Accuracy of identification following a manual selection and what the stimuli meant were determined by responses to a series of verbally presented categorizing clues or occasionally clues presented as a printed list for visual inspection by the right hemisphere. Previous experience with these subjects had established that reliable 'yes–no' answers could be elicited in response to questions about left visual field, right-hemisphere registered stimuli. To illustrate this procedure, the following is an excerpt from one of the tests conducted on L.B. (Sperry *et al.* 1979: 159–60).

Test A. Subject was shown an array of four pictures of people, singly and in groups. Three of the pictures contained unknowns and one in the upper left included a picture of Hitler in uniform standing with four other men. L.B. was asked to point to 'any of these that you recognize'.

L.B.   Examined the card for approximately 14 seconds and then pointed to the face of Hitler.

Ex.   'Do you recognize that one? Is that the only one?'

L.B.   Again inspected the full array but did not point to any others.

Ex.   'Well, on this: is this one a "thumbs-up" or a "thumbs-down" item for you?'

L.B.   Signalled 'thumbs-down'.

Ex.   'That's another "thumbs-down"?'

L.B.   'Guess I'm antisocial.' (Because this was the third consecutive 'thumbs-down'.)

Ex.   'Who is it?'

L.B.   'GI came to mind. I mean...' Subject at this point was seen to be tracing letters with the first finger of the left

	hand on the back of his right hand.
Ex.	'You're writing with your left hand; let's keep the cues out.'
L.B.	'Sorry about that.'
Ex.	'Is it someone you know personally... or from entertainment... or historical, or... ?'
L.B.	Interrupted and said 'Historical'.
Ex.	Recent or... ?'
L.B.	'Past.'
Ex.	'This country or another country?'
L.B.	'Another country, I think.'
Ex.	'Prime minister, king, president... any of them?'
L.B.	'Gee,' and pondered with accompanying lip movements for several seconds.
Ex.	Giving further cues: 'Great Britain?... Germany... ?'
L.B.	Interrupted and said definitively 'Germany' and then after a slight pause added – 'Hitler'.

The researchers interpreted this study as follows. L.B.'s right hemisphere readily identified the picture of Hitler and did not recognize any others. The left hemisphere, cued by the mental aura generated by the picture and by the response of the right hemisphere to the examiner's questions, guessed 'government' and 'historical' while rejecting alternatives like a personal acquaintance or someone in entertainment.[12] The continuing vagueness of the (left) speaking hemisphere's orientation was illustrated by its hesitancy along with comments like, 'Another country, I think'. The accurate identification in the 'mute' hemisphere was indicated in the negative responses to the series of false vocal cues and the immediate, firm positive response to 'Germany' followed shortly by vocal confirmation of the correct identification of Hitler.

As a result of this and other tests conducted on L.B. and the subject N.B., it was concluded that, at a level comparable to that of the left hemisphere of the same subject, the right hemisphere possessed a well-developed sense of self and social awareness. The kinds of emotional reactions that were generated and the selectivity of the response to follow-up questions of the examiners and to the vocal cues from the subject's own comments, showed that true identifications were made by the right hemisphere accompanied by appropriate cognitive and conative associations.

2.6   THE LATERALIZATION OF SOUND

As we saw briefly in chapter 1, the results of Kimura's incipient
dichotic listening tests indicated a right-ear/left-hemisphere advantage in both normal and brain-damaged subjects in tasks
involving the ability to understand and produce speech. Subsequent tests conducted by Kimura and others largely confirm this
result (Kimura 1967; Kimura and Folb 1968; Milner *et al.* 1968;
Springer and Gazzaniga 1975; Gordon 1980).

Having found a right-ear advantage for the perception of dichotically presented speech stimuli, Kimura searched for tasks that
could lead to a left-ear advantage and therefore right-hemisphere
superiority. By 1964 she reported such an effect in the perception
of melodic excerpts. Her study consisted of dichotically presenting
two 4-second excerpts from chamber music to normal subjects, immediately after which four melodies, two of which had just been
dichotically presented, were binaurally presented in succession.
Kimura found a left-ear advantage in this task. (Subsequent dichotic listening research indicated that in certain cases the
left-ear/right-hemisphere advantage for music can be affected by
the musical experience of the subject. Bever and Chiarello (1974)
reported a right-hemisphere advantage in non-musicians but a left-
hemisphere advantage in musicians. Noting this result, Gaede *et
al.* (1978) proposed that musical aptitude rather than experience
is the relevant factor in determining the shifts to a left-hemisphere
advantage in music.)[13]

The left-ear, right-hemisphere advantage for music has been
found applicable to other paralinguistic phenomena. Curry (1967)
reported a left-ear effect for dichotically presented environmental
sounds such as a car starting, toilet flushing and tooth brushing.
King and Kimura (1972) complemented this finding by reporting
a left-ear advantage for vocal non-speech sounds such as laughing,
sighing, and crying.

In 1980, Jakobson gave a lecture at New York University in
which he ventured, 'a tentative answer to the question of the
general criteria which separates the two spheres of auditory stimuli
from each other – those processed by the left and those processed
by the right hemispheres of the brain' (Jakobson 1980: 15). This
lecture is significant because Jakobson draws his conclusions from
neuropsychological sources in the form of dichotic listening, evidence from commissurotomized and brain-lesioned subjects, and

the use of electroshocks to understand the respective processing modes of the hemispheres. On the role played by the right hemisphere in processing non-speech sounds, Jakobson concluded:

> Those sound phenomena which demand an unimpaired functioning of the right hemisphere all have in common one noticeable trait: they display a direct, immediate, ostensive relation between their external, material form and what is signalled. Our perception of speech sounds demands an apprehension of the sound pattern and of its cognitive function in a given language, whereas the identification of any non-speech sound requires an immediate recognition of the stimulus perceived, its identification in form and meaning.
>
> (Jakobson 1980: 19)

We are presented with examples of the type of sound processed by the right hemisphere: sharpening a pencil, yawning, singing birds, splashing water, neighing horses, thunder peals, clanking metal, barking dogs, and so forth. (For a complete list of the examples, see pp. 19–21; for some of their sources, see Knox and Kimura 1970; King and Kimura 1972; Balonov and Deglin 1977.) It is noted further that during the right hemisphere's inactivation the sound of applause has been taken for the winnowing of grain, laughter for crying, a thunderstorm for engine noise and a dog barking for cackling hens (21).

Regarding speech, Jakobson concludes that the right hemisphere plays the dominant role in intoning sentences, so that, 'In the period of the right hemisphere's inactivation the identification of intonations sharply worsens' (26–27). It is also concluded that the right hemisphere secures the subject's ability to identify an acquaintance's voice in their visual absence (with an inactivated right hemisphere subjects failed to recognize the most familiar of voices). Further, with the right hemisphere inactive, the subject cannot trace the source and direction of the voice, 'Thus the spatial hearing remains unaltered after left-sided shocks but appears disturbed after right-sided ones' (28).

In summary we find Jakobson concluding, 'The chief ability of the right hemisphere in handling auditory percepts is their immediate change into a simple, concrete concept lying outside of language proper, disclosing the nearest contiguous source of the sound stimulus produced and heard' (28).

Regarding the right hemisphere's ability to deal with concrete concepts, there is now a great deal of evidence to suggest that it plays a significant role in processing high imagery words and in providing an existentially related context in which language can operate. For a significant review of this field, see Perecman (1983).

2.7 OTHER NEUROPSYCHOLOGICAL EVIDENCE

We saw in chapter 1 how Galin and Ornstein (1972), using EEG monitoring techniques, showed a link between the right hemisphere and the capacity to process spatially oriented information. Buschbaum and Fedio (1970) observed differences in evoked potential (EP) while normal subjects viewed verbal and non-verbal stimuli tachistoscopically presented to the respective visual fields. The verbal presentations consisted of three-letter words, the non-verbal presentations of nonsense stimuli composed of an artificial alphabet of letters. When recordings were made from the occipital lobes, results showed greater differences between the EPs to the two types of stimuli in the left hemisphere compared to the right. Cohn (1971) recorded EPs from the respective hemispheres while subjects were presented with simple stimuli such as clicks or blank flashes of light. It was found that the right hemisphere dominated in processing this class of stimuli. For a review of the application of EEG and related brain monitoring procedures, see Thatcher *et al.* (1983).

In keeping with the majority of results from neuropsychology, those from eye movement studies indicate that the right hemisphere dominates in processing spatially oriented information. Gur and Gur (1977a) tested 49 normal male students by asking them a series of 'spatially oriented' and 'linguistically oriented' questions. For example, a subject was asked to explain a linguistically oriented proverb of the order: Rome was not built in a day. He was subsequently asked to answer a spatially oriented question of the order: Visualize sitting in front of a typewriter and attempt to reconstruct the relative positions of F and B. When asking such questions the examiner sat directly behind the subject. After results were tabulated from a hidden video camera, it was found that subjects' eyes moved to the right 64 per cent of the time when answering linguistically oriented questions yet only 31 per cent of the time when answering spatially oriented ones.

The experiment was repeated with the examiner sitting directly in front of the subject. When answering questions in this situation the subjects' eyes moved consistently either to the left or right regardless of the type of question asked. From this result it was proposed that the stress of having to face an authoritative figure (the examiner) demanded that subjects had to rely more exclusively on the hemisphere habitually used in everyday circumstances.

The results of the subjects' habitual eye movements were tabulated and subjects accordingly classified as 'left-movers', 'bidirectionals', or 'right-movers'. The results were subsequently correlated with the study area researched by any one subject. The correlation showed that 'right-movers' tended to specialize in science subjects, 'left-movers' in the humanities, and the 'bidirectionals' fell somewhere to the centre of the two extremes. Further similar tests were performed by Gur and Gur (1977b) on 28 right-handed males. Results of these tests confirmed the researchers' original findings.

It is worth noting in conclusion that an experiment similar to those conducted by Gur and Gur had been constructed by Schwartz *et al.* (1975) at Harvard University. Results showed that the spatial and emotional content of questions are additive in their proclivity to engage the right hemisphere whereas questions that are either spatial or emotional are less likely to engage this hemisphere.

Chapter Three

THE POSSIBLE ORIGINS OF CEREBRAL SPECIALIZATION

3.1 INTRODUCTION

There is a great deal of evidence to suggest that hemispheric differences, both anatomical and functional, are innately determined and become reinforced with the development of the neonate. In this chapter I therefore review data relevant to the phylogeny and ontogeny of the brain on the assumption that this perspective can illuminate the behaviour it produces in the modern adult, including our relations to symbol systems found in the culture. This is the final chapter to concentrate on presenting neuropsychologically related evidence; in contrast to my two opening chapters, however, in this one I draw independent conclusions thereby setting the pattern for all subsequent chapters.

3.2 THE PHYLOGENY OF CEREBRAL SPECIALIZATION

The view that cerebral specialization of function is innately determined, and therefore present at birth, is substantiated by observations of the brain's anatomy, as indicated by Dimond:

> From the time of the earliest observations it has also been noted that the asymmetries are present in the brains of foetuses and the newborn. They therefore precede early environmental experience and it is extremely unlikely, therefore, that they occur as a result of experience.

> (Dimond 1979: 194)

We are informed that in the Chapel aux Saints Neanderthal man skull (c. 30,000BC) the imprint of Sylvian fissures is visible on both sides. The imprint on the right side is angled up more sharply, however, indicating that cerebral asymmetry was anatomically present early on in our prehistory. Dimond's speculations are substantiated by the research of Galaburda *et al.* when they propose:

> Structural asymmetries between the hemispheres are found in the human brain. Asymmetries in the auditory regions and in the Sylvian fissures are present even in the fetus. The Sylvian asymmetries may have also existed in Neanderthal man... Thus, the striking auditory asymmetries could underlie language lateralization. The asymmetries in the frontal and occipital lobes and the lateral ventricles are correlated to hand preference.
>
> (Galaburda *et al.* 1978: 852)

Remaining with the theme of the possible origins of cerebral specialization, I shall now turn to the research of Alexander Marshack (1976) who has made a lifetime study of prehistorical artifacts. The paper of concern here resulted from the availability of animal statuettes produced by Neanderthals (c. 30,000BC) and discovered in the Vogelherd, Southern Germany. Using the artifacts as basic data, Marshack draws conclusions which he argues are relevant to an understanding of the evolved human capacity for symbol marking and language and which can help to explain how bilateral symmetry gave way to bilateral specialization.

Careful analysis of the artifacts showed evidence of long-term use and symbol marking thereby implying that they had been employed in a number of different ways and in different contexts. In a horse statuette, for example, the stone is unrealistically marked with a series of zigzags, multiple arcs, and smaller strokes suggesting that, 'One class of symbol is used with another class as a part of a complex, interrelated, traditional usage' (276). It is further proposed that the marks suggest a sequential, cumulative notation indicative of an incipient form of language.

Similar conclusions are drawn regarding an engraved rib, microscopic analysis of which showed that, 'the image had been made sequentially as a series of connected, festooned double arcs, beginning at left and ending at right with a multiple marking' (278). It is again proposed that a symbolic use is implied indicating a cognitive capacity for abstraction, modelling, and manufacture of a different order that can be deduced from the subsistence tool industries. In general it is argued that the artifacts:

> were not tools made for practical use or in order to make

other tools but were instead part of a sequence and strategy which was 'non-adaptive' except in a cultural context. The engraved artifacts pose an even more intriguing problem since they suggest the presence of a tradition of non-representational symbolic marking that may have required some form of 'linguistic' explanation.

(Marshack 1976: 277)

Marshack continues by suggesting that the manufacture of the artifacts in fact probably formed an intrinsic part of Neanderthals' evolving language capacity. He speculates that when manufacturing an artifact the Neanderthal artisan probably used the right hand to hold the cutting tool to shape the image while the left hand held the material, adjusting it for purposes of orientation, judging it for weight and size, and so forth. In this way the right hand formed a particular class of image which, although non-linguistic, was related to naming.[1] It was not, therefore, only the manipulative capacity of the hominid hand as a tool-user that was involved but a two-handed competence with a highly evolved right-handed, vision-oriented specialization for symbol-forming, aided by the left hand supplying a different form of input. It is proposed that this two-handed competence:

has relevance for lateralization, cerebral dominance, cross-modal association, etc., but involved also are such 'modes' or aspects as motivation, planning, cognitive modelling, symbolic sequencing, and an exceedingly fine acuity in the kinesthetic, somesthetic and visual inputs.

Marshack speculates further on:

One must explore the possibility that visually oriented 'two-handedness' of the human type, with all of its cross-modal neurological correlates, evolved in conjunction with an increasingly lateralized, corticalized capacity for vocal communication.

(Marshack: 1976: 280)

It is speculated further that the eye-hand relationship required to manufacture symbolic artifacts was probably also involved in the more general cultural differentiation of classes according to their presence in different contexts. Early humans thus probably evolved a gestural system capable of denoting whether a type of wood was usable or not, an insect edible or not, a snake dangerous or not, and so forth. The relationship would probably also have been involved in some type of terrain 'modelling' with indications of place and direction performed by pointing. In general, the eye-hand relationship would have become increasingly involved in complex, specialized, and often cultural or 'learned' skills.

From this it follows that the emerging capacity to communicate through the use of gestural signs would have evolved in conjunction with a cognitive system with the potential for internally relevant iconic signing. (In other words, before early humans could communicate information about their environment through the use of a gestural syntax, it would have been necessary for the brain to have become sufficiently 'hardwired' to adequately process the system.)[2]

Marshack continues by proposing that, concomitant with the development of gestural syntax, would have developed the capacity to modulate the 'vocal–auditory' call system because this would improve the gestural system by lending it affect. For example, whereas a hand gesture could denote 'snake' and perhaps indicate its size and direction, a concurrent modulation of the fear call could indicate if it were dangerous. In this way, the vocal-auditory system complemented the eye-hand gestural system and the former developed into a formalized speech system. (From this it follows, given the clinical data, that speech eventually became lateralized to the left hemisphere.)

Overall, then, Marshack constructs a model primarily concerned with the phylogenetic emergence of speech and language involving the dominant use of the right hand which complements Gazzaniga's views on the ontogenetic emergence of language, as we shall see presently.

Importantly, however, associations of the vocal-auditory class in early humans could have eventually 'overlapped' with the implication that the eye-hand gestural system became increasingly redundant.

The specific vocalization accompanying a signing for serpent ... could itself become a sign for the class. Once instituted as a functional mode, such specifying affect vocalization could function at a distance in time and space from the object. It would thus become an abstracted, non-iconic symbol and, though originally of limbic derivation, it could now serve, proto-linguistically, in a symbolically structured situation with a lessened affect.

(Marshack 1976: 281)

It is nonetheless emphasized that, being volitional, such modulated vocalization would have required association with the eye-hand gestural signing system – in fact it could function only by referring to this system because, without it, vocalization would have had little communication value. From this it follows that language, and possibly other non-linguistic communication systems, developed as a consequence of the association of two or more classes of sensory information.[3] Even so, as language developed in humans it did, of course, become capable of functioning autonomously, that is, without overt reference to the eye-hand gestural system.

3.3 DAVID MARR'S RESEARCH ON VISION

I shall now introduce aspects of Marr's research on vision (1982). Because one of his assumptions is that our visual system developed as a result of our goal-oriented needs as a species, it complements Marshack's evolutionary perspective on cerebral specialization.[4] There is an additional strong neuropsychological element in Marr's research. This is found both in his general interest in the relations between the brain and vision and in Warrington and Taylor's observations of how lesions to the respective hemispheres affect the capacity to process certain classes of visual information.

Warrington and Taylor's research indicated that subjects with right- hemisphere damage experienced no difficulty in identifying water buckets and similar objects in side views, yet were unable to identify them from above. A group of left-hemisphere damaged subjects readily identified objects from both views, however (Warrington and Taylor 1973). Later investigations confirmed these initial results (Warrington and Taylor 1978). This research suggested to Marr that the brain stores information about the use and function of objects separately from information about their shape, and that our visual system permits us to recognize objects even when we cannot describe their function.

Marr noted that those parts of a visual image that we name and that have a meaning for us do not necessarily possess visually distinctive characteristics that can be uniquely specified in a computer program. For example, the same circle could represent a wheel, the sun, or a table-top, contingent upon the context of the situation. From such observations he went on to ask which are the important features for seeing an object and which can be ignored. He approached this problem by (a) proposing that the visual system is goal-oriented, and (b) proposing that it can be broken down into a number of capacities or 'modules'.

Regarding the first proposal, Marr observed that the frog's visual system is adapted to identify food in the form of small moving specks (flies); the fly's system is adapted to identify a surface on which to land, and so forth.[5] Because higher animals, including humans, spend (or spent) much of their time in motion gathering food, one of the major functions of our visual system is to be able to readily identify three-dimensional objects so that they can be either avoided or manipulated. From this Marr reasoned that only after we have understood the goals of the visual system (which he called 'level one' of understanding) are we in a position to study the procedures or 'programs' it uses to achieve them (called 'level two' of understanding). He also distinguished a third level of understanding a visual system which refers to its 'hardware', that is, neurons or electric circuits in which the procedures on level two can be effected.

Regarding the proposal that the visual system is modular, Marr argued that vision consists of a number of relatively independent subtasks that can be studied in isolation which he called the *principle of modular design*. For example, recognizing an object and realizing its three dimensionality could depend on the activation of different and independent modules. Marr thus reasoned that our mental ability to accomplish tasks is solved by processing independent problems that constitute the general task. If this were not so, new mental capacities that developed in the course of evolution would have had to develop in perfect form in unison. From an evolutionary perspective modular design is important, because:

> if a process is not designed in this way, a small change in one place has consequences in many other places. As a result, the process as a whole is extremely difficult to debug or to improve, whether by a human designer or in the course of natural evolution, because a small change to improve one part has to be accompanied by many simultaneous, compensatory changes elsewhere. The principle of modular design does not forbid weak interactions between different modules

in a task but it does insist that the overall organization must, to a first approximation, be modular.

(Marr 1982: 102)

From his two fundamental proposals Marr constructed a model of the different types of symbolic representations necessary for the visual system in humans to be able to compute the everyday, three-dimensional world. He argued that in the first stages of visual processing the brain computes a two-dimensional sketch, termed the *primal sketch*, from the variation in light intensities, termed the *grey level image*, that fall on the retinal surfaces. The brain derives the primal sketch by noting where the level of greyness changes on the retina relayed by some 160 million light receptors sensitive to varying levels of illumination. (It may be useful to conceptualize this process in terms of how a monochromatic photograph is constructed.)

The lines constituting the primal sketch represent the extent, magnitude (thickness of line) and direction of the changes. What is visually significant about an object usually occurs where the illumination changes, particularly along its edges where there are significant variations in its surface texture (cf. Kennedy 1974: 132). Marr proposed that this initial computation is automatic, although if the symbol derived from the primal sketch is unfamiliar to us, other more complex modules related to memory may be activated.

From the primal sketch is derived the 2½-D sketch which indicates to the brain that the primal sketch has three dimensions. A number of independent calculations or modules are required to form this new symbol, including an automatic analysis of separate effects such as shading, motion, shape, and so forth. However, the 2½-D sketch only informs the brain about an object seen from a fixed perspective point, it does not give a full sense of the object in space which requires a new set of computations.

In order for the brain to compute a generalized view of an object in space, termed the 3-D model, it attempts to determine if there is a line which, if 'drawn through' the 2½-D sketch, establishes its basic pattern of symmetry. This line is termed either the *principal axis* or the principle line of symmetry.[6] Having established the principal axis, the brain then proceeds to search for further relevant symmetrical branching lines. For example, human beings have a principal axis running through the head and body, and other branching lines of symmetry running through arms, legs, fingers, toes, and so forth. Marr suggested that stick figures of mammals constructed from pipe cleaners, although offering a minimum of visual information, make sense to us because they propose basic lines of symmetry that resemble the lines the brain in fact computes.[7] The principal axis therefore suggests to us our general description of objects while the finer distinguishing details are concluded from an analysis of the branching lines of symmetry.

Having established an object's principal and related branching axes, the brain subsequently 'fills them out' by transposing the contours it has already derived from the 2½-D sketch onto the various axes of symmetry thereby producing the complete 3-D model.

The relevance the principal axis plays in everyday visual perception was thus illustrated by Warrington and Taylor's right-hemisphere brain damaged subjects who experienced difficulty in recognizing objects with their principal axes foreshortened.

I return to both Marshack and Marr's research in my conclusion to this chapter when I show how it can help to account for the possible origins of cerebral specialization. For the present I shall review evidence relevant to the ontogeny of cerebral specialization.

3.4 THE ONTOGENY OF CEREBRAL SPECIALIZATION

As is the case with the majority of mammals, at birth the human brain is underdeveloped and undergoes rapid structural and functional maturation in infancy and early childhood.[8] For example, the brain grows physically and as this occurs its neural connections multiply rapidly; insulating fatty layers called myelin develop around nerve fibres making them more effective conductors of electrical impulses. The myelination process is particularly relevant to early cerebral lateralization when it is taken into account that, due to its lack of myelination, the hemispheres' major communication pathway, the corpus callosum, is not yet functional. Certain authorities propose that its myelination is incomplete until puberty (Lennenberg 1967; Yakolev and LeCours 1967), others that the process is essentially complete by the age of five or six (Basser 1962; Witelson 1977).

The fact that the corpus callosum is not functional at birth has the significant corollary that the neonate is effectively a 'natural' split-brain subject with certain implications, as Gazzaniga (1970) points out: 'there is at least suggestive evidence that the human neonate is a split-brain for a good period of time, and is thus subject to a special class of phenomena that is not apparent in the non-split-brain' (131). Gazzaniga proposes that the corpus callosum becomes functionally 'hooked up' at approximately two years of age and then goes on to speculate that, prior to this time, 'When the child was set to explore with the right hand, visual, auditory, or tactual engrams would be established in the left hemisphere. The same would be true for a left hand set with the engrams being laid down on the right' (131).

Gazzaniga continues by proposing that, because the majority of children explore using primarily their right hand, the left hemisphere soon becomes more developed than the right (taking into account the X functional mode). It would therefore soon know more and consequently ask more questions which increasingly become 'read out' as a right-hand activity. Hand use thus reinforces hemisphere use with the result that the two systems mutually reinforce each other in a circular fashion. Because of its right-hand advantage, therefore, the left hemisphere becomes more proficient at any one stage of early hemispheric development with this proficiency increasing over time.[9]

It is reasoned that consistent with this view is the prediction that the functionally disconnected right hemisphere would develop a separate language system when the child manipulated the environment using its left hand. It is emphasized that this fits the neurological data in that left-hemisphere lesions in the young child do not cause a total language disruption as is the case in the adult (with the corollary that the right hemisphere initially possesses some language competence). When the corpus callosum becomes myelinated to the point where everything experienced by one hemisphere is instantly communicated to the other, a different logic emerges, however, particularly regarding memory. The dominant left hemisphere attends to external information and, while receiving and processing it, the right hemisphere is held disengaged. In this way, duplication of engrams and learning in general would become less frequent with the result that the left hemisphere increasingly dominates in most tasks. Increasingly, right-hemisphere possessed information becomes redundant and might eventually become lost, erased, or functionally suppressed. Gazzaniga concludes:

In summary, the view is that some evidence exists that the young child has a partially split-brain. It would therefore be subject to a certain class of phenomena which, in the main, would encourage or enhance lateral development of language.

(Gazzaniga 1970: 134)

Gazzaniga therefore argues that at birth the right hemisphere may possess some language potential, thereby implying an initial plasticity of function, but in the majority of cases this potential is suppressed by the left hemisphere whose dominance is reinforced by right-hand use.

It should be emphasized, however, that the clinical data from Broca's research onwards logically implies that in spite of some initial cerebral plasticity of function, it so happens that our species' language potential is primarily left-hemisphere localized. From this it follows that a major weakness in the 'right-hand stimulating and reinforcing left-hemisphere dominance for language' argument is that it fails to explain the emergence of right-hand dominance in the first instance.

3.5 STUDIES OF THE INFANT AND CHILD BRAIN

The view that the brain is genetically programmed at birth to process different types of information and that plasticity is limited in degree, is clearly substantiated by the neuropsychological data. A number of tests have been carried out to determine the development of hemispheric specialization in infants and children, all of which indicate that specialization is innately determined.

Dennis and Whitaker (1976) studied three 9- to 10-year-old hemispherectomy operation subjects, all of whom had been operated on before 5 months of age. One subject was a right-hemispherectomy subject, the others had had the left hemisphere removed. Results of the studies showed that discrimination and articulation of speech sounds were normal in all three children and all were equally competent at producing and discriminating between words. However, significant differences between hemispheric competence occurred in tests designed to elicit the subjects' ability to deal with syntax. For example, each child was asked to judge the acceptability of the following passive sentences:

1. I paid the money by the man.
2. I was paid the money to the lady.
3. I was paid the money by the boy.

The right-hemispherectomy, left-hemisphere intact subject correctly indicated that sentences 1 and 2 are grammatically incorrect and sentence 3 is acceptable. The two left-hemispherectomy subjects failed to make these distinctions – in other words, they thought all three sentences to be grammatically correct.

From this result it was concluded that the right-hemispherectomy subjects failed to accurately comprehend the meaning of passive sentences. Further tests led to the conclusion that the right-hemispherectomy defect is an organizational, analytic and syntactical problem rather than one rooted in the conceptual or semantic aspects of language. These conclusions indicate that cerebral plasticity of function is limited in the infant brain thereby substantiating the view that asymmetries between the hemispheres are present at birth.

This view is reinforced by tests performed on normal infants. Turkewitz (1977) monitored the direction in which 100 healthy babies held their heads while lying on their backs. He found that for 88 per cent of the time a right direction predominated thereby implying left-hemisphere dominance. Kinsbourne (1978) repeated this experiment and arrived at similar conclusions. Kinsbourne has argued elsewhere (1975) that cerebral specialization is complete in its essentials at birth.

Both dichotic listening and electrophysiological recording techniques have been used to study hemispheric specialization in normal infants and children. Entus (1977) adapted the dichotic listening technique so that it could be applied to infants by encouraging them to suck on a nipple to receive dichotic listening presentations of word pairs. Each time the infant sucked with a previously specified force, the same words were presented. This procedure continued until the infants habituated to the dichotic pair as evidenced by a sustained reduction in the sucking rate. At this point, either the left- or right-ear stimulus was changed and the examiner monitored the infants for changes in the sucking rate. The results of this study indicated that the infants noticed a change in either ear, that is, the sucking rate increased, but a change in the right ear produced a greater increase in sucking. From this it follows that a right-ear, left-hemisphere advantage for words exists in the infant brain which is innately determined.

The Entus result corroborates results of an experiment conducted by Molfese *et al.* two years previously, when the researchers found evidence of asymmetries in the electrical recordings of the respective hemispheres in the infant. Speech sounds such as 'ba' were presented to infants from approximately 1 week to 10 months while EP activity was recorded from both hemispheres. It was found that responses of greater amplitude, implying greater mental involvement in sound-processing, came from the left hemisphere in 9 of the 10 infants tested. When the infants were presented with certain non-speech sounds, however, an opposite effect was obtained – all 10 infants exhibited EPs of a greater amplitude in the right hemisphere. A later study by Molfese (1977) constructed along similar lines confirmed these results. (These results complement Kimura's model, reviewed in chapters 1 and 2.)

Wada and Davis (1977) recorded the EP to clicks and flashes of light and subsequently measured the coherence, that is, similarity of forms, of the EP in the temporal and occipital regions of the infant brain. This test was influenced by the researchers' earlier work with adult subjects tested with sodium amytal. Results showed that coherence was largest for clicks in the left (speech) hemisphere and for flashes of light in the right (non-speech) hemisphere. Similar results were found in their study of 50 infants ranging from 1 day to 5 weeks. Findings indicated that occipital and temporal lobe forms of response to clicks were of greater similarity within the left hemisphere than within the right, whereas similarity moved toward the right hemisphere when flashes were presented. It was concluded that these results reflect hemispheric specialization and that specialization is present at birth.

Although the results of these infant studies are not conclusive they are nonetheless significant because they suggest that, although the neonate may not be properly conscious of the nature of the experimental stimuli being presented, localized parts of the brain are innately equipped to specialize in processing certain classes of information.

3.6   PERSONAL CONCLUSIONS

In this conclusion I develop a hypothesis that can help illuminate the nature and origins of cerebral specialization in the modern adult. I shall begin by arguing that important correlations exist between the research of Marshack and Marr.

The conclusions Marshack draws from his analysis of the Vogelherd statuettes implies that by this stage in prehistory our species had evolved a certain level of consciousness. That is, if the artifacts are seen as a symptom of our emerging capacity to abstract and conceptualize, it must have developed concomitant with our capacity to rationalize both our environment and personal status. This in turn suggests a degree of self-awareness and an emerging capacity to differentiate ourselves as a species. Exactly what the artifacts denoted or symbolized, or why they were manufactured in the first instance, will probably never be fully known. They nonetheless imply that significant correlations existed between our emerging capacity to represent our sensorily derived experience of the world through iconic imagery and a capacity to say something about the world through the use of arbitrary symbol forms symptomatic of a protolanguage.

This view that these two symbol forms were integrally related is phenomenally substantiated by the fact that Neanderthals chose to superimpose their protolinguistic message directly onto their iconic one, that is, marks on the statuettes. This relationship is also implied by the supposition that the manufacture of both symbol forms involved the use of common sense modalities. That is, the eye-hand relationship employed to carve iconic imagery into a statuette was also involved in carving its protolinguistic markings.

These observable and implied neurological correlations indicate the following sequence. The iconic image, carved from stone or bone and a reminder of phenomena, provided a cultural (and visual) context which facilitated our emerging capacity to abstract our experiences of phenomena through the intervention of arbitrary symbolic markings. Therefore, unlike the blank page on which we now write, a direct visual and causal relation existed between the protolanguage and its subject. That is: subject (phenomenal world) becomes → iconic image (visual reminder of phenomena) becomes → subject for protolanguage.

(I am not arguing that Neanderthals found it necessary to first construct an iconic equivalent – the horse statuette, for example – of a subject before they could verbalize their relations to it. What seems more likely is that the act of visually and sensibly constructing an equivalent helped to cognitively clarify its referent's separate existence thereby facilitating its verbalization. A similar visual-verbal relationship is often observable in children's drawing. For example, a picture may be drawn of a church, bells ringing, which is accompanied by the words 'ding-dong' written 'onto' or near the church. I return to the significance of such visual-verbal relations in children's drawing in chapter 5.)

The relationship between the iconic and the arbitrary is also suggested by the implied mental operations involved in Marshack's view of our emerging gestural system. For example, the capacity to gesturally denote the presence of a snake, perhaps by the undulatory motion of an arm or hand, implies the use of both forms. That is, the motion must have served as a quasi-iconic reminder of our visually derived understanding of snake movements and also been capable of abstractly denoting something about the species thereby implying the potential to name and classify things in the world.

As the eye-hand gestural system developed, however, it became redundant because the modulated vocal-auditory system that accompanied it developed into speech proper. With the development of speech our species became capable of recalling and cognitively manipulating the phenomenal world in its absence without overt recourse to the gestural system. This must have afforded us the distinct advantage of being able to plan our actions. The speech and language capacity in general increasingly pervaded our evolving cognitive system and, given the clinical data, became lateralized to the left hemisphere.

Importantly, however, although iconic symbol forming and the eye-hand system in general may have become redundant to verbalization, these systems nonetheless continued to develop independently. This is surely evidenced by the discoveries made in painting and sculpture throughout the history of art – given that these art forms imply the capacity for sophisticated iconic symbol forming through the use of the eye-hand system. This argument has the possible and important corollary that the left hemisphere's preoccupation with language functions facilitated the right hemisphere's potential to develop unique non-linguistic and yet intelligent capacities, perhaps once shared by the left hemisphere, of an iconic and phenomenally related class. The neuropsychological researchers Springer and Deutsch imply views similar to my own when they speculate:

Just as the left hemisphere evolved language, a symbol system surpassing any single sense modality, perhaps areas of the right hemisphere evolved ways of presenting abstractly two- and three-dimensional relationships of the external world grasped through vision, touch and movement.

(Springer and Deutsch 1981: 202)

It is reasoned from this that our ability to generate mental maps, rotate images, and conceptualize mechanical contraptions, could very well be an abstract, internalized right-brain counterpart to the motor skills of the left brain (202).

From what I have so far hypothesized, the following pattern can be seen as emerging.

1 Our species differentiates itself and the phenomenal world by representing the world through the manufacture of iconic imagery. The imagery implies the use of a spatio-temporal cognitive strategy currently associated with the right hemisphere. The phenomenal world has something said about it in its absence.

2 Superimposed directly onto the iconic imagery, sequentially oriented protolinguistic marks implying a conceptualization and abstraction both of the imagery and its referent together with a linguistic potential currently associated with the left hemisphere. The imagery, as a reminder of the phenomenal world in its absence, has something said about it in its presence.

3 The eye-hand system, used in the manufacture of the imagery, its protolinguistic marks and the gestural system, is complemented by our evolving capacity to modulate the vocal-auditory system. Speech proper eventually develops thereby enabling the world to be abstractly manipulated in its phenomenal absence.

4 The language and speech capacities eventually become 'hardwired' to the left hemisphere thereby facilitating the right hemisphere's potential to develop non-linguistic capacities of a spatially oriented and iconic class. These capacities become 'hardwired' to the right hemisphere.

5 The phylogenetic evolution of the brain affects its ontogenetic development. Thus the significance of the data indicating that hemispheric differences are innately determined and the

general indications that the left hemisphere specializes in processing linguistic information whereas the right hemisphere specializes in processing visual information.

Drawing from the research of both Marr and Warrington and Taylor, I shall now develop the argument that bilateral specialization evolved to the point where it became capable of effecting a dualistic response to perception.

If bilateral specialization is related to the clinical data that right-hemisphere intact subjects experienced no difficulty in recognizing objects with foreshortened axes, whereas this was not the case with right-hemisphere damaged subjects, this suggests the following possibility. Affected by its evolving language capacity, the left hemisphere increasingly became programmed to process information adopting an abstracting and conceptualizing mode of operation. So pervasive was this occurrence in the left hemisphere that it affected the way in which all inputted or relayed information, including visual information, was processed – thus the left hemisphere's incapacity to process objects viewed from oblique angles.

This hypothesis concurs in general with Marr's principle of modular design which states that evolutionary changes that occurred in one part of the brain need not have been accompanied by simultaneous, compensatory changes elsewhere. Therefore, any changes that occurred in the left hemisphere (around the areas of Broca or Wernicke, for example) to affect its mode of information-processing, need not have occurred in its partner hemisphere. Thereafter, any changes that occurred in the right hemisphere (around the parietal lobe, for example) to affect its mode of information-processing, need not have occurred in its partner hemisphere, and so forth.

Taking into account Warrington and Taylor's research, from this it follows that the modularized component necessary to the visual system's capacity to interpret objects with foreshortened axes, became lateralized to the right hemisphere.[10] This conclusion concurs with the clinical data which indicates in general that the right hemisphere dominates in processing most classes of spatially oriented information. It also makes common sense from an evolutionary perspective that early on parts of our visual system were goal-oriented in such a way as to have been capable of processing all kinds of objects, regardless of their axes' orientations, for purely pragmatic reasons. For example, the Neanderthal hunter surely had to be capable of identifying a dangerous species of animal from any angle in order to survive. Further, this process surely had to be instant, automatic, and intuitive simply because, as a body moves in space in front of us, or we in front of it, or both, its principal and related branching axes change millisecond by millisecond.

Nonetheless, while the research of both Marr and Warrington and Taylor implies that the right hemisphere dominates in processing spatially oriented information, it does not imply that the left hemisphere is entirely redundant in this regard. Warrington and Taylor's right-hemisphere damaged subjects managed to identify objects without foreshortened axes.

I shall now develop a hypothesis to account for this (limited) left-hemisphere capacity which complements my original one that bilateral specialization is capable of effecting a dualistic response to perception.

It seems to me that one of the essential reasons why an object without a foreshortened principal axis is more readily left (language) hemisphere identifiable is because in this position the object can usually be identified by its shape alone. That is, the shape becomes, in a propositional manner, a sign for the object's class. In terms of linguistically identifying or naming the object, no further information of a three-dimensional class is required. In fact, with their principal axes apparent, most objects, particularly if they are symmetrical, can be identified by their shapes provided that these have become sufficiently culturally (and neurologically) encoded so as to typify what they represent. In this way, a number of visual symbols found in *The Highway Code* or at international conferences, while partially resembling their referents, essentially function as quasi-iconic indicators that are 'read' as a part of a quasi-language system. Further, this form of indicator can often be developed into a visual 'syntax' by adding wholly arbitrary symbolic codes.[11]

To illustrate this point I constructed three shapes of a well-known object (Figure 5). When it is viewed from a perspective that foreshortens its principal axis, its resulting shape (a) is at best ambiguous. When the object is viewed from a perspective that makes its principal axis apparent, its resulting shape (b) is easily recognizable and nameable. When the shape is viewed from position b, but with an arbitrary 'X' shape added (c), its b shape is easily read as a part of a quasi-visual syntax. In this last example we do not

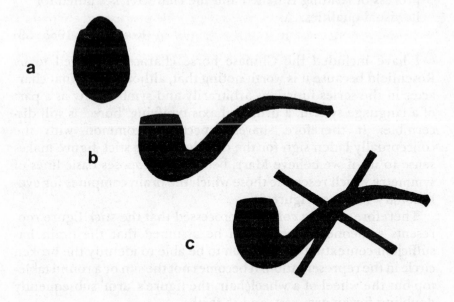

Figure 5   Pipes in silhouette

perceive the new shape as a strange-looking pipe with five stems, we perceive it as *No Smoking*.

A possible corollary from this is that when objects are exclusively viewed from appropriate 'symbolic' or 'generic' angles, they are more likely to activate a left-hemisphere associated, conceptually laden, and language oriented *reading* strategy. In fact I would go further and argue that objects viewed from 'generic' angles share a great deal in common with pictographs in ancient Egyptian hieroglyphics and certain Chinese ideograms. And here we can refer to the views of Rosenfield:

> A picture understood as a picture is deciphered by the visual system; a picture used in writing is ultimately deciphered by the language centres. Pictures used in writing represent very different kinds of information from pictures used in drawing. The brain makes the distinction depending on what kind of information it is trying to derive from the visual information. When reading the Chinese character for a horse, no-one *sees* that the character vaguely resembles a horse unless the

process of reading is halted and the character is studied for
its visual qualities.

(Rosenfield 1985: 53)

I have included the Chinese horse character referred to by
Rosenfield because it is worth noting that, although the final character in the series functions arbitrarily and symbolically as a part
of a language system, a principal axis typifying 'horse' is still dis-
cernible. It therefore shares aspects in common with the
conceptually laden sign for the disabled whose stick figure makes
sense to us, if we believe Marr, because it proposes basic lines of
symmetry which resemble those which the brain computes for evolutionary reasons (Figure 6).

Therefore, having correctly processed that the stick figure represents someone sitting, it can be assumed that the brain has
sufficient contextual information to be able to identify the broken
circle in the representation. It becomes not the sun or a round table-
top but the wheel of a wheelchair, the figure's 'arm' subsequently
doubling for an arm rest, and so forth.

Importantly from a neurological perspective, Rosenfield informs

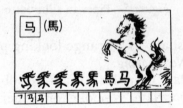

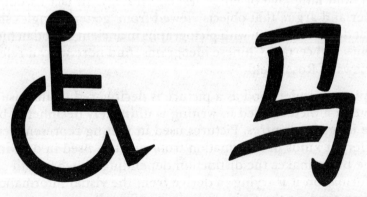

Figure 6   Chinese horse character and sign for the disabled

us that recent clinical data suggests that pictographs or ideograms are unrelated to drawings. In relation to Chinese ideographs (kanji), for example, and phonetic symbols (kana), studies show that the classical left hemisphere areas of Broca and Wernicke must be intact to read both forms (53).

This clearly relates to Warrington and Taylor's observations that left-hemisphere intact subjects experienced no difficulty in recognizing an object provided it was viewed from the necessary 'generic' angle. The general implication is that the left hemisphere specializes in processing visual information primarily of an arbitrary or quasi-iconic propositionally oriented class which has meaning only as a part of a sequentially oriented and symbolic language system. From this it could follow that brain-damaged subjects with only the left hemisphere intact – and therefore without the mediating force of the right hemisphere's mode of processing – should tend towards processing *all* types of visual information adopting a propositional, language oriented cognitive strategy. This view is substantiated by Gardner's observations of right-hemisphere damaged subjects whose drawings reveal, 'an almost exclusive dependence upon propositional knowledge regarding the object (the names of the features of that object) rather than sensitivity to the actually perceived contours of the entities and of the parts to be depicted' (Gardner 1984: 182).

3.7   CONCLUDING REMARKS

Drawing from neuropsychologically related evidence, I have argued in this chapter that, such was the path of evolution, bilateral specialization is innately determined and therefore present at birth (with the corollary assumption that the respective hemispheres are genetically programmed to process distinct types of information). From this it follows that it is not simply the sense modality through which information is relayed to the brain that dictates which hemisphere will be dominantly activated when engaged in a particular task. For example, information that activates a dominantly right-hemisphere response may be relayed to the brain via the visual, auditory or other modal systems, or a cross-modal combination of several systems.

This is relevant to my *compatibility proposition*, found in the introduction to this book, which stated: if the respective hemispheres possess qualitatively different modes of cognitive processing it is a reasonable assumption that these developed for some good evolutionary reasons which carry over, as it were, to affect the way in which symbol systems and information generally found in the culture are processed. From this it follows that certain forms of symbolic stimuli are more likely to elicit, and therefore be compatible with, particular modes of cognitive processing while inhibiting others.

Chapter Four

THE RIGHT-HEMISPHERE COGNITIVE PARADIGM

4.1 INTRODUCTION

I concluded the last chapter by proposing that the respective hemispheres are genetically programmed at birth to process different types of information regardless of which sense modality relays the information to the brain. In this chapter I investigate more fully the nature and implications of the right-hemisphere associated cognitive paradigm and show its relevance to picture perception. Because, in addition to drawing from new material to support my views, I do this by referring to the data introduced over the last three chapters, I shall first briefly review the type of information the right hemisphere specializes in processing.

Regarding information associated with the visual system, we have seen that the right hemisphere dominates in recognizing faces (Hecaen and Angelergues 1962; Hecaen and Sauguet 1971; Levy *et al.* 1972); in processing objects viewed from unconventional angles (Warrington and Taylor 1973); in processing spatially oriented information synthetically (Nebes 1972, 1973); in drawing (Bogen 1969a); in maze learning (Kimura 1963), and can respond to pictorial stimuli through the use of manipulospatial strategies (Nebes, 1972; Gazzaniga and Le Doux 1978; Sperry et al. 1979).

We have also seen that the right hemisphere dominates in processing certain types of paralinguistic auditory phenomena. For example, its propensity to process non-speech sounds of a general class (King and Kimura 1972; Molfese *et al.* 1975; Entus 1977); musical sounds (Kimura 1964), and environmental sounds (Curry 1967; Jakobson 1980).

More generally, we have seen that the right hemisphere specializes in processing spatially oriented information regardless of the sense modality through which the information is perceived

(Buschbaum and Fedio 1970; Galin and Ornstein 1972; Schwartz *et al.* 1975; Gur and Gur 1977a, 1977b).

4.2 THE AUTOMATIC, INTUITIVE, AND SPATIALLY ORIENTED NATURE OF THE RIGHT-HEMISPHERE PARADIGM

The right hemisphere dominates in facial recognition. In everyday circumstances this perceptual and implied mental capacity is clearly automatic, intuitive, and does not need to be learned. When searching for a familiar face in a crowd we do not have to logically deduce, adopting a step-by-step cognitive strategy, its visual-spatial identity *vis-à-vis* all other visually perceived facial configurations. When searching for the face of a friend we do not ask ourselves in a propositional manner: how far apart are their eyebrows, the shape of their nose, the prominence of their chin, and so forth. Rather, we search for and perhaps eventually identify the familiar face adopting what can for the present be described as an holistic cognitive mode.

It is also worth noting regarding the conclusions I drew from Warrington and Taylor's paper (1973) that not only facial recognition but recognition of spatial configurations in general is typically automatically accomplished regardless of the angle from which an object is visually perceived. That is, we are typically capable of instantly recognizing an object from a wide variety of unconventional views.

Regarding the Kimura study (1964), it is also true that we exhibit a capacity to automatically perceive and intuitively respond to music regardless of its cultural and historical origin. This does not assume that some learned knowledge, perhaps imparted through language, of a piece of music's origin cannot affect our response. We are nonetheless capable of expressing like or dislike, interest or disinterest, for the piece on hearing it for the first time (cf. Pateman 1986).

Jakobson's conclusion that those sound phenomena demanding an unimpaired functioning of the right hemisphere all display in common a direct, immediate, and ostensive relationship between their material form and what is signalled, also indicates an automatic, intuitive, existential, and spatially oriented right-hemisphere paradigm. For example, a 'barking' sound not only automatically suggests the existence of a dog but also its approximate position in space relative to our own. A different sound indicates that a train is approaching perhaps to the left, an aeroplane is passing overhead, and so forth. In such situations we do not ask ourselves in a propositional manner: is this sound produced by a mechanical or animal agency; what type of machine or species does it derive from; from where in space is the sound coming.[1]

The extent to which the spatially oriented task of drawing (Bogen 1969a) or maze learning (Kimura 1963) is a predominantly automatic and intuitive process is more problematic. Certainly the capacity to accomplish both activities can appear to be primarily automatic and intuitive – for example, watching a skilled artist effortlessly draw a subject. Nonetheless, the capacity to draw is clearly enhanced by certain forms of tuition which develop relatively propositionally oriented strategies. In fact, it can be reasonably argued that many of the important advances made in perspective at the Renaissance were greatly influenced by carefully learned formal skills handed down from master to pupil.

Picture production should be clearly distinguished from picture perception, however. The capacity to produce a picture, by other than mechanical means, should not be confused with the capacity to perceive and respond to pictures.[2] We no more require the skills of a Michaelangelo to perceive and appreciate his Sistine chapel ceiling than we require the skills of a Beethoven to appreciate one of his symphonies.[3] As Kennedy succinctly states regarding picture perception, 'To make pictures is an art, but recognition of depictions is largely a gift the environment and nature allows us gratis' (Kennedy 1974: 155). I examine theories of picture perception in chapter 6.

4.3 INTERSENSORIAL PERCEPTION, MEMORY, AND THE RIGHT HEMISPHERE[4]

In this section I argue that the right hemisphere exhibits the capacity to make intelligent connections between intersensorially perceived information and relating it to knowledge stored in memory.

In the Nebes' study (1972) we saw that the subject was required to manually examine three geometric designs, hidden from view, while looking at a sketch of one of the designs presented in fragmented form. The task was to determine which of the examined designs matched the sketch. The result that in the majority of cases the right hemisphere managed to successfully accomplish this task (whereas, it should be emphasized, the left hemisphere did not) clearly indicates that it is capable of linking and cognizing different types of non-linguistic and intersensorially perceived information.

Regarding my associated contention that the right hemisphere can relate sensorily perceived information to memory data, I shall first turn to Jakobson's conclusion, reviewed in chapter 2, that, 'the chief ability of the right hemisphere in handling auditory percepts is their immediate change into a simple concrete concept lying outside of language proper'. In order to change an auditory percept into a simple concrete concept, it has to be assumed that *extra*-auditory components of the concept, stored in memory, contribute to its realization. Therefore, if we hear 'barking' we intuitively know that it signifies the existence of a dog. Put differently, the aurally perceived stimulus 'triggers' our originally visually perceived understanding, stored in memory, of what dogs in general *look like*. In this way, auditory information perceived in the present, is capable of triggering, in a cross-modal fashion, information perceived in the past through a different sense modality, the visual system.

This is not to assume that 'barking' automatically conjures a precise mental image of a St Bernard or a corgi, although if we happen to be particularly familiar with dogs this is more likely to be the case. Nonetheless, distinct 'barkings' tend to suggest more than a vague notion of 'dogginess'. Life experience dictates our associations and expectations in such a way that on hearing a high-pitched yapping from around a corner we would be surprised if a St Bernard came into view.

In advance of Jakobson's conclusion that the right hemisphere exhibits the capacity to change an auditory percept into a single concrete concept, the results of the Gazzaniga and Ledoux tests on P.S., reviewed in chapter 2, imply that it is capable of changing percepts into *multiple* concepts. That is, P.S.'s capacity to match two visually perceived forms, the snow scene and the shovel, suggests the following.

P.S.'s right-hemisphere perception of the snow scene, complete with house, car, and snowman, prompted memory traces of the right hemisphere's originally intersensorially perceived under-

standing of the scene including its affective connotations, associations, implied concepts, and so forth. For example, that snow is
cold and pleasant or unpleasant, that it possesses a certain texture,
that it can or cannot be manually manipulated, that snow-covered
houses with smoke from the chimney suggest fire, warmth, and
human habitation, that a car possesses wheels enabling it to move,
that snow-surrounded cars have difficulty in moving, and so forth
through an infinitesimal series of permutations. It also has to be
assumed that similar associations and connotations applied to *all*
of the images in the choice array presented to P.S.: the lawnmower,
brush, shovel, pick, apple, electric toaster, hammer, and chicken
head (Figure 4). From this miscellany P.S. chose just one item to
match the snow scene – the shovel.

In order to make this correct choice it can be hypothesized that,
triggered by its visual perception of the snow scene, P.S.'s right
hemisphere first reviewed the scene's multiple permutations and
implied concepts. Subsequently both hemispheres, triggered by
their visual perceptions of the choice array images viewed in free
vision, reviewed the images' multiple permutations and implied
concepts. Finally, P.S.'s right hemisphere independently concluded that one particular concept from the snow scene's
permutations and one concept from the choice array of images
were most compatible. That is, the shovel, as a manually operated
tool capable of clearing substances, contextualized the possibility
that some of the snow, probably surrounding the car or house,
needed clearing.[5] It seems to me, then, that P.S.'s overall right-
hemisphere response to the initially visually perceived information
was highly complex and intelligent, as implied by schema 2.

Schema 2

Visually perceived information, i.e. snow scene, lawnmower,
brush, shovel, pick, apple, toaster, hammer, chicken head →
triggers → originally intersensorially perceived memory data
→ triggers → related affective associations, expectations and
concepts that are cognized to produce → decision denoted in
the form of a manually signified response, i.e. P.S.'s left hand
points to shovel.

It is reasonable to assume that an approximately similar associative process occurred regarding the subject L.B., examined by

Sperry *et al.* (1979), reviewed in chapter 2. Thus, L.B. managed to successfully identify a photograph of Hitler from a choice array of typically unfamiliar images and affectively respond to his choice.

What is particularly interesting about this test is that, by verbally prompting L.B., the examiners afford us some insight into the nature of the right hemisphere's subjective memory mechanisms. For example, that his right hemisphere signalled a *dislike* of Hitler by a 'thumbs-down' response; that it was capable of contextualizing Hitler as being someone historical as distinct from the other possibilities involved; or that it probably did not perceive Hitler as being a prime minister, king, or president because of his commonly acknowledged status as a dictator.

4.4   AMODAL CONTROL MECHANISMS

In this section I introduce Fodor's general view on mental organization and then show how it has specific implications for right-hemisphere function.

Fodor (1983) argues convincingly that our mental structures are related to *transducers, input systems,* and *central systems.*

Transducers more or less represent the five senses. Input systems, which relate to information inputted through the senses, are *modular* and suppose *vertical* faculties, that is, each faculty is isolated from the next. A modular system deals with only one type of information (they are domain specific) so that the aural input system will exclusively compute incoming sound, the visual input system exclusively compute the visual characteristics of an object, and so forth. (This view complements both Marr and Warrington and Taylor's research reviewed in chapter 3.)

In this way, modules are limited because they can draw from only a specific range of information *encapsulated* in the module. The point of information encapsulation is that it allows for speedy information processing thereby enabling a fast identification of stimuli. Input systems therefore transduce information in such a way as to allow real world phenomena to become accessible at speed to mental systems.

Central systems do not specialize in processing only certain types of information but function as 'central intelligence areas' that, when necessary, 'correct' information once it has passed through the input systems. We thus find Fodor proposing, 'the representations that input systems deliver have to interface somewhere and the computational mechanisms that effect the interface must *ipso facto* have access to information from more than one cognitive domain' (1983: 101–2).

Fodor's hypothesis is that input systems, initially activated by one or more sensory transducers (visual, auditory, olfactory, etc.) draw certain conclusions based upon mentally encoded but limited knowledge. Because input systems are vertical and cannot communicate with each other, however, and because they work at speed and are not open to introspection, they sometimes need to refer to a less specialized bank of knowledge as represented by the central systems. In this way, central systems 'look simultaneously at the representations delivered by the various input systems and at the information in memory, and they arrive at the best (i.e. best available) hypothesis about how the world must be' (102).

One of the major functions of central systems is to avoid 'wishful thinking'. It is argued that our relations to the world usually occur after perceptual integration: we tend to think (central systems) before we act. That is, because input systems are selective (they encapsulate information) and because they work at speed, they are not always reliable so that we are sometimes deceived by our perceptions. Information passing through the input systems therefore often needs to confer with the central intelligence areas which then make appropriate 'believed' corrections, a process described as the *fixation of perceptual belief*.[6]

The implied complexity of the mental processes that enabled both P.S. and L.B. to (successfully) respond to sophisticated visual stimuli, indicates that the right hemisphere is capable of higher modes of cognitive processing without the mediation of the classic language centres (given that neither subject's right hemisphere had access to these centres because of their commissurotomies). Further, the subjects' capacity to successfully respond implies the existence of a right-hemisphere, sensory transcendent or *amodal control mechanism* (ACM) capable of synthesizing and drawing intelligent conclusions from intersensorially perceived information in the light of memory data. That is, if my view on the associative processes which led to both P.S. and L.B.'s correct choices is correct, then they surely had to refer to a right hemisphere ACM simply because the multiple permutations triggered by the initially visually perceived information was surely too heavy a load to be processed by (in Fodor's terms, encapsulated by) the visual system alone.

The implication in the Nebes' study (1972) that the subject managed to relate and successfully act upon information perceived through the visual and touch modalities, also indicates the existence of a right-hemisphere ACM capable of intelligently understanding and responding to intersensorially perceived information and information stored in memory.

A right-hemisphere ACM is also indicated from the conclusions I reached in the light of those of Jakobson (1980). Thus the implication that the right hemisphere can relate aurally perceived information to relevant memory data, conceptualize the information and, when necessary, act upon it. On hearing a ferocious barking from around the corner it may not only be associated with a potentially dangerous dog but also prepare us for action.

4.5   AMODAL CONTROL MECHANISMS ARE LATERALIZED

In this section I contend that the respective hemispheres possess distinct ACMs and that the dominant system in the left hemisphere is, in effect, the language centres.

My proposal that P.S. referred exclusively to his right-hemisphere ACM when making his 'shovel' choice, raises several important issues regarding our beliefs being fixated by central intelligence areas. By P.S. making this choice it is a reasonable assumption that, after looking at the various representations delivered by the visual system and at its memory data, the right hemisphere arrived at the best possible hypothesis, namely, that shovels can be associated with clearing snow. So far, Fodor's fixation of perceptual belief holds good in regard to the right hemisphere. It also holds good for the left hemisphere possessing fixing systems, as evidenced by P.S.'s capacity to arrive at a correct conclusion regarding the connection between chicken claws and chicken heads.

In the case of P.S., however, we are not talking about *one* overriding system capable of fixating beliefs but *two* or possibly more systems capable of simultaneously operating in his brain. From this it follows that we are referring to a minimum of two input systems associated with vision, two independent banks of memory data, and so forth (see chapter 3.6 and section 6 of my introduction to this book). This is important because it could follow that P.S. possesses a lateralized or even divided consciousness. We are certainly talking about P.S. possessing two mental systems capable of fixating beliefs because, due to his split-brain condition, two hemispherically independent choices were made regarding the initially visually inputted stimuli.

This has as a possible corollary that in the cerebrally intact individual both hemispheres either possess, or potentially possess, fixating systems capable of making higher order decisions without the direct intervention of the partner hemisphere.[7] Further, in the case of P.S., his left hemisphere not only made the correct choice (chicken claw/head) but also exhibited the tendency to construct – and to all effects believe in – an incorrect hypothesis simply because it lacked sufficient information to arrive at a correct one. This was evidenced by his confabulation, 'I saw a claw and I picked the chicken, and you have to clean out the chicken shed with a shovel'.

Although this confabulation based around shovels and imagined chicken sheds was plainly 'wrong', it does not necessarily contradict Fodor's hypothesis that fixating central systems exist in the brain which reach reasoned conclusions by drawing from encapsulated information and memory data. It can thus be assumed that P.S.'s left-hemisphere based central system or ACM made the correct chicken/head choice and also observed the right hemisphere's overt behaviour in the form of his left hand pointing to the shovel. At this stage, while lacking the vital fourth, it nonetheless possessed three units of information from which to construct a best (best available) hypothesis as to why the shovel had been chosen, namely, chicken claws, chicken heads and shovels.[8]

What is significant about P.S.'s confabulation is the left hemisphere mechanism that produced it did not acknowledge it simply possessed insufficient information to say why a shovel had been chosen from the choice array of items; instead attempts were made to verbally qualify and rationalize the situation. Thus the relevance of Gazzaniga and LeDoux's conclusion that it is as if the verbal self looks out and sees what a person is doing and from that knowledge it interprets a reality.

This does not mean that P.S.'s left hemisphere chicken claw/head choice was necessarily exclusively linguistically governed or organized. His left-hemisphere propensity to verbally confabulate with certainty as to the reason for his right-hemisphere choice in the light of its own, does, however, imply that the left hemisphere's dominant and overriding ACM is linguistically governed. Given the clinical data, it follows that it can be located around the classic language centres of Broca and Wernicke. (This view is consistent with the one I introduced in chapter 3 which proposed that so pervasive was the development of language in the left hemisphere that it affected the way in which all inputted information was processed, including that class perceived by the visual modality. I return to the significance of the left hemisphere's tendency to dominate, particularly regarding linguistic descriptions of the representational visual image, in later chapters.)

If my interpretation of Fodor's fixation of perceptual belief hypothesis in the light of my interpretation of P.S.'s observed behaviour is correct, while it may not seriously undermine the hypothetical existence of central systems, it does call into question their functional value. That is, if central systems are dualistically or even pluralistically represented in the brain, this has as a possible corollary that the brain has two or more belief systems potentially capable of mutually conflicting in response to certain types of stimuli. This raises the important question: which system are we to believe in?

It could be argued that no definitive answer exists to this question because it so happens that we are (paradoxically) capable of many beliefs, some of which mutually conflict (cf. Festinger 1957). A more positive answer, however, might be that belief systems do not normally conflict because the one employed is typically the most appropriate to the situation experienced. From this it could follow that the brain as a whole possesses a 'master' cognitive mechanism capable of in most, but not in all, instances occluding the intervention of inappropriate fixating systems.

4.6   ACMS AND ACLMS

I have argued that the right hemisphere dominates in automatically and intuitively processing information, perceived in particular through the visual and auditory modalities, and derived from non-linguistic, spatially oriented and concrete sources.

These facets suppose the existence of a type of ACM which, as an integral part of our biological organism as a whole, evolved so

as to be capable of intelligently but intuitively coping with information from the phenomenal world as it instantly unfolds, even
when the information is under-determined. This form of coping
in turn implies the existence of a cognitive strategy which processes
information so that its significance is determined by an holistic understanding of phenomena. For example, on hearing a ferocious
'barking' we tend to instantly derive an overall grasp of the situation thereby implying the possession of an ACM capable of
synthesizing the initial stimulus (barking) in the light of our whole
experience and related expectations of the phenomenon. We do
not, therefore, respond to the sound as if it were a singular and
arbitrary sound percept disembodied from its referent.

In fact, so strong is our holistic yet under-determined understanding of certain classes of existentially derived phenomena, that
certain *iconic* stimuli forms (images, paralinguistic sounds, etc.)
which reproduce only aspects of the phenomena, can lead to a kind
of perceptual paradox. That is, the iconic stimuli can induce in us
existentially derived response tendencies in spite of our better
knowledge as to the phenomenal unreality of the stimuli.

For example, we find it difficult to psychologically divorce certain auditory percepts from their holistically related and concretely
derived concepts, even when fully aware that only the auditory percept exists. On hearing 'barking' on a sound effects record, and we
are fully aware that no dog is phenomenally present, we find it
difficult to disassociate the percept from our holistic understanding
of, and possible response to, its concrete referent, in this (hypothetical) case, a certain kind of dog in a certain kind of mood. A similar
process may be seen as applying to our perceptions of certain iconic
visual stimuli forms, as we shall see in section 4.7 and further on
in this book.

For the present I shall introduce the views of Dreyfus (1972) who,
in his critique of artificial intelligence, proposes biologically involved reasons for why it is that we are capable of using an
under-determined (holistic) expectation to organize our experience.

Adopting an essentially phenomenological approach, Dreyfus
argues that the 'higher' determinate, logical, and detached forms
of human intelligence are necessarily derived from and guided by
global and complicated 'lower' forms. It is our bodily skills that enable us not only to recognize objects in each sense modality, but

by a felt equivalence of our exploratory skills, we can see and touch the same object. In order for a computer to do the same thing it would have to be programmed to make a specific list of characteristics of a visually analysed object and compare the list of recorded traits by moving tactile receptors over the same object. This means that there would need to exist an 'internal' model of each object in each (artificial) sense modality and that the recognition of an object seen and felt would have to pass through the analysis of that object in terms of common features.

However, unlike computers, our biological status enables us to bypass this type of formal analysis. A human skill, unlike a set of fixed responses, can be brought to bear in an indefinite number of ways so that when someone acquires a skill he:

> does not weld together individual movements and individual stimuli but acquires the power to respond with a certain type of solution to situations of a certain general form. The situations may differ widely from place to place, and the response movements may be entrusted sometimes to one operative organ, sometimes to another, both situations and responses in the various cases having in common not so much a partial identity of elements as a shared significance.
>
> (Dreyfus 1972: 161)

Dreyfus thus emphasizes that our higher cognitions of the phenomenal world often rely upon our biological status. It is this condition that allows information to be shared among our sensory systems (and our mental faculties) and it is our capacity to correlate this information which lends it significance. It is pointed out that we can recognize a rough surface with our hands, our feet, or even our gaze.[9] Our bodies are therefore what Merleau-Ponty calls a 'synergic system', that is, 'a ready-made system of equivalents and transpositions from one sense to another' (Dreyfus 1972: 161).

It is concluded that the advantage of this system is that the body can constantly modify its expectations in terms of a more flexible criterion: as *embodied* we find it unnecessary to check for specific characteristics but simply for whether, on the basis of our expectations, we are coping with a situation. Coping need not be defined by any specific set of traits, however, but by an ongoing mastery that Merleau-Ponty describes as *maximum grasp*. What counts as maximum grasp varies with the goal of the agent and the resources of the situation so that it cannot be expressed in situation or purpose-free situations.

There are several points argued by Dreyfus that, when collectively viewed, provide an attractive description of the nature and functions of the right-hemisphere ACM (although it is fair to point out that Dreyfus' sources do not include neuropsychology).

First, his argument that by a felt equivalence of our bodily skills (our five senses, Fodor's *transducers*, Piaget's intersensorial perception, etc.) we can see and touch the same object, complements my own that the right hemisphere is capable of relating intersensorially and primarily non-linguistically perceived information. Second, his argument that it is our capacity to relate information shared among our senses that lends it *significance*, agrees with my own that the right hemisphere possesses an ACM capable of independently correlating and *intelligently* responding to intersensorially perceived information in the light of information stored in memory. Third, his argument that it is our capacity to make sense of shared information which allows us to modify our expectations, concurs with my own that the right hemisphere possesses an ACM capable of automatically and intuitively coping with information from the phenomenal world as it instantly unfolds.

Although our 'higher' forms of cognition may be derived from and guided by global and involved 'lower' (bodily-mediated) forms, it should be emphasized that I am not arguing that our capacity to register sensorily inputted information is the exclusive role of the right hemisphere. Clearly both hemispheres are capable of registering and exchanging knowledge in some form as evidenced by the X functional mode.

Neither am I arguing that our capacity to cognize sensorily and intersensorially perceived information of a non-linguistic origin is the exclusive prerogative of the right hemisphere. Our capacity to formulate, conceptualize, and abstractly manipulate our experience of the world through the filter system of language argues against this possibility. In fact, Dreyfus sees our biological status as playing an important a role in language construction, and particularly performance, as it plays regarding any other human activity.

But there exists an important distinction between first linguistically formulating sensorily perceived information and responding to it, and responding to the information without first linguistically formulating it. The former process implies that information can be abstracted and rationalized thereby allowing it to be manipulated in its phenomenal absence. As I indicated in chapter 3, this must have afforded Neanderthals the distinct advantage of being able to plan their actions. The latter process, however, which in neuropsychological terms implies that certain forms of incoming information *bypass* the language centres, also implies that it can be more directly and intuitively processed.

With certain reservations, therefore, I wish to contend that intuiting is a way of describing *our right-hemisphere associated capacity to circumvent formal linguistic analysis by directly relating to certain types of incoming information*. In terms of hemispheric ACMs, the distinction between these implied 'rationalizing' and 'intuiting' modes becomes more obvious when a left-hemisphere *amodal control language mechanism* (ACLM) is introduced into my arguments to produce schema 3.

Schema 3

LH processed information → ACM → ACLM → response
RH processed information → ACM → response

This argument that certain types of information bypass the language centres is substantiated by Gazzaniga's recent modular view of mental activity.[10] Drawing from his lateralization research, Gazzaniga proposes that much of the brain is organized into relatively independent functioning units that work in parallel. The brain is therefore not an indivisible whole operating in a single way to solve all problems; rather, there exist many specific and identifiably distinct units which deal with the information they are exposed to from both the human and external environment. Further, these modular activities:

> frequently operate apart from our conscious verbal selves.
> That does not mean that they are 'unconscious' or 'preconscious' processes and outside our capacity to isolate and understand them. Rather, they are processes going on in parallel to our conscious thought, and contributing to our conscious structure in identifiable ways.
>
> (Gazzaniga 1985: 4)

If Gazzaniga is right in arguing that certain mental activities operate apart from our verbal selves, this does not mean that this self readily acknowledges this, as Dimond indicates in the following sceptical argument:

> Language immediately makes a claim for itself to be prince among the mental processes, and to be the exclusive medium of mental function, denying often by its existence the presence of other modes of thought. The primacy of language as perceived through its own system is, I believe, responsible for the creation of two fundamental illusions. The first of these concerns the production of an illusory self. This production is on a level with the phenomenon so well known in other circles as an active structuring of experience. The second illusion is that of the essential unity of the individual. All the evidence suggests that the brain must analyse at many levels and that its mental activity is composed of different parts, and yet whenever one argues about mental pluralism and the importance of the multi-layered approach, the fact is that the brain fails to recognize this and remains dominated by the unified strand of its own subjective experience.
>
> (Dimond 1979: 216)[11]

This view that language fails to recognize other (non-linguistic) modes of processing, clearly relates to my *translation and causation issues*, introduced in section 2 of my introduction to this book. That is, the question of the extent to which language can plausibly explicate the representational visual image, and if it cannot, what is it which, regardless, continues to motivate its use by visual-art related hermeneutic disciplines. I return to these issues in chapters 6 and 7. For the present I shall attempt to show that significant relations exist between right-hemisphere associated modes of processing and picture perception.

4.7   THE RIGHT HEMISPHERE AND PICTURE PERCEPTION

I have argued that the right hemisphere possesses an ACM which specializes in intuitively (without the intervention of the language centres) responding to certain types of spatially involved and phenomenally derived information, even when the information is under-determined. From this it does not follow that the exclusive use of this ACM is to enable us to cope with the vicissitudes of the unfolding world (although I suggest that this was the major reason for its evolution).

In fact, to insist upon this view would be to contradict at least some of what has so far been been indicated. For example, we saw in the Nebes' study (1972) that subjects exhibited a dominantly right-hemisphere capacity to make intelligent connections between iconic and manually perceived information (a sketch of a geometric design and the three-dimensional geometric designs themselves). We saw in the Gazzaniga and LeDoux study (1978) that P.S. also exhibited a right-hemisphere capacity to make intelligent connections between iconic imagery presented in the form of a snow scene, lawnmower, brush, shovel, and so forth. Similarly, in the Sperry *et al.* study (1979), L.B. exhibited a right-hemisphere capacity to affectively respond to a picture of Hitler chosen from a choice array of images. Results of the Levy *et al.* study (1972) indicated that the right hemisphere dominated in recognizing (tachistoscopically presented) chimeric faces and other miscellaneous chimeric imagery forms, and so forth.

Sketches of geometric designs, tachistoscopically presented images, and pictures of snow scenes and Hitler, although derived from phenomenal sources, cannot be construed as phenomenal entities, with the implication that they are incapable of unfolding in any phenomenal sense and therefore do not require the same form of coping as might be associated with their phenomenal referents.[12]

Nonetheless, if we take into account the results of the tests conducted on P.S. and L.B. (and many similar results are well-documented), there exist good grounds for supposing that iconic images 'covertly' unfold because of their potential to remind us of the nature of our *holistic* relations to the phenomenal world. Put differently, I am suggesting that, although iconic images necessarily present us with exclusively visual and therefore underdetermined information *vis-à-vis* their referents, this is sufficient to elicit memory associations and relevant response tendencies, derived from our intersensorially (and not therefore exclusively visually) mediated understanding of their phenomenal referents. If this were not the case, it would be difficult to explain how P.S.'s right hemisphere managed to make intelligent and *practically* oriented connections between an *image* of a snow scene and a shovel.

I shall therefore conclude this chapter by introducing what

might be termed a neuropsychologically substantiated theory of picture perception. It agues that *the same right-hemisphere paradigm which evolved to enable us to cope with certain classes of information derived from the phenomenal world, has become sufficiently mentally 'hardwired' that it can be activated in its entirety on encountering the world's visual representation.* Therefore, although pictures are not phenomenal entities *per se*, as visually-spatially involved *r*epresentations of phenomena, they can activate right-hemisphere ACM, ACLM bypassing ways of processing information that, although of a 'higher' cognitive order, are derived from and guided by 'lower' sensorily/bodily mediated forms of knowledge.

This theory of picture perception is consistent with the view I presented in the introduction to this book and developed in chapter 3.6. That is, if the respective hemispheres possess qualitatively different modes of cognitive processing, it is a reasonable assumption that these developed for some good evolutionary reasons which 'carry over' to affect the way in which symbol forms found in the culture are processed. I qualify my theory from a developmental perspective in the next chapter when relating it to children's drawing. For the present refer to schema 4.

Schema 4

Visual marks activate → visual-spatial memory systems containing experientially derived visual information → automatically reconstitutes marks into visual representation of world → memory banks containing additional sensorily derived information relevant to representation leads to it becoming → a representation with an existential life → activates → further associations, expectations and response tendencies.

In this way, as iconic representations, pictures can elicit traces of our intersensorially mediated and dominantly right-hemisphere processed understanding of the phenomenal world in all its complexity. Consequently, although under-determined, pictures transcend their purely visually encapsulated meaning.

Chapter Five

CHILDREN'S DRAWING

5.1 INTRODUCTION

I concluded the last chapter by arguing that, as iconic representations, pictures can elicit traces of our intersensorially mediated knowledge of the world in all its complexity. The meaning of pictures is therefore reliant upon more than our knowledge of the world as we perceive it reduced to a two-dimensional image. Because this view is unlikely to go unchallenged, however, and because it is central to my later arguments, I substantiate and develop it over the next two chapters. These are concerned with the nature of picture production, perception and response and should be viewed as important preludes to the theory of aesthetic response I develop in chapter 7.

In this chapter I argue that we can learn a great deal about adult picture perception by referring to the time when we spontaneously produced pictures as an integral part of our life development; that is, to when we were children and picture-making represented a unique means of expressing what the unfolding, intersensorially mediated world meant to us.

I shall begin by reviewing some of Piaget's views on child development. These are relevant to my arguments because of their emphasis that children's visual perception is not to be understood in isolation as it functions as an integral part of their 'heterogeneous schemata'. Drawing is therefore not a merely passive visual recording of the world but consequent upon events being (holistically) participated in by the child. Piaget's views are of a more general relevance because, in keeping with my own research strategy, they employ mentalistic concepts that have a biological and genetic explanation for their development.

5.2   PIAGET AND INTERSENSORIAL PERCEPTION

Piaget argues that from the beginning of the infant's orientations in looking, coordinations exist between vision and hearing and subsequently between vision and sucking and finally between vision and prehension, touch and kinesthetic impressions. It is argued further, that: 'These intersensorial coordinations, this organization of heterogeneous schemata will give the visual images increasingly rich meaning and make visual assimilation no longer an end in itself but an instrument of vaster assimilations' (1966: 75).

By the time the child has reached 7 or 8 months, unknown objects are looked at in order to *act*, that is, to enable the child to assimilate the new object to the separate schemata of weighing, friction, falling, and so forth. Each separate schemata is not isolated from the next, however, because there is no longer only organization inside visual schemata but between those and all others, and it is this progressive organization, 'which endows the visual images with their meaning and solidifies them in inserting them in a total universe' (76).

Therefore, although the organization of visual schemata forms a closed totality so that vision constitutes a value system in itself (something akin to Fodor's vertical and encapsulating *input systems*), the visual schemata are coordinated to other schemata where there exists reciprocal organization and adaption. In this way, visual assimilation becomes a simple means at the service of higher ends and therefore a value derived in relation to *principal values*. Principal values are constituted by the totalities pertaining to hearing, prehension, and the activities they generate. (Principal values therefore share aspects in common with Fodor's 'pooling' *central systems* and my *ACMs*).

The general development of children occurs neither exclusively as a result of their naturally unfolding cognitive maturation nor exclusively as a result of external environmental factors. Rather, both 'nature' and 'nurture' play their role in child development:

> the input, the stimulus, is filtered through a structure that consists of the action schemes (or at a higher level, the operations of thought) which in turn are modified and enriched when the subject's behavioural repertoire is accommodated to the demands of reality; the filtering of the input is called *assimilation*; the modification of the internal schemes to fit

89

reality is called *accommodation*.

(Piaget and Inhelder 1969: 6)[1]

This reciprocal relationship between reality and action schemes, symptomatic of the *sensori-motor period*, eventually leads to children's capacity to internalize relationships and culminates in a sudden comprehension or insight symptomatic of the *semiotic period*. At this stage in children's development they become capable of summoning and manipulating aspects of the phenomenal world in its absence. One of the unique ways in which this is done is through drawing, an intermediate stage between symbolic play and the mental image, and an act which reinforces the transition from representation in action to representation in thought.[2]

Symbolic play is essentially that stage when children become capable of *pretending* to act in a certain way, including using their bodies as a symbolic vehicle. In all cases, says Piaget, the representation is obvious (pretending to sleep, for example) and the signifier is an imitative gesture although accompanied by objects that are becoming symbolic.

Symbolic play functions partially as an escape mechanism whereby children, constantly obliged to adapt themselves to an adult and still physically alien world, attempt to assimilate reality without the typical coercions and sanctions. Therefore, although the symbols used in play are borrowed from imitation, they are not used to 'accurately' picture reality but constitute a 'symbolic language' that can be developed by the self and is capable of being modified according to present needs. Symbolic play is therefore described as, 'The creation of symbols at will in order to express everything in the child's life experience that cannot be formulated and assimilated by the means of language alone' (Piaget and Inhelder 1969: 61).

Mental images, problematic because of their internalization, are generally described as holistically constituted. (Mental images are therefore no more direct visual copies of the world than are Saussure's sound images direct auditory copies of the pure acoustic blast. Cf. Saussure 1983.) Piaget suggests that the reason for this discrepancy between pure visual perception and mental images is because an imagined body movement is accompanied by the same pattern of electrical waves, whether cortical or muscular, as when a movement is physically accomplished in real life. Also, if the mental image were merely a prolongation of pure visual perception it should appear from birth, yet it only occurs at the semiotic period.[3] Mental images are therefore active copies of perceptual data consequent upon events in the world being participated in by the child. From this conclusion Piaget reasons:

> there can be no perception that is not incorporated in a complex sensori-motor activity. A perception linked to a particular centration is only a kind of snapshot or *still*, cut off from the dynamic flow of perceptual activity which reacts constantly upon the perceptions on which it is based and which it links together.
>
> (Piaget and Inhelder 1956: 39)

It is argued elsewhere that adults as well as children need mental images because they too need a system of signifiers capable of dealing with, 'the whole past perceptual experience of the subject' (Piaget and Inhelder 1969: 70).

Both symbolic play and mental images are therefore on the whole extra-linguistically constituted and serve relatively general functions. That is, symbolic play expresses everything that cannot be formulated and assimilated by language alone, and the mental image deals with the whole past perceptual experience of the individual.

From this it follows that if drawing lies somewhere between symbolic play and the mental image, it must also be initially concerned with everything that cannot be formulated by language alone. Piaget nonetheless argues that even in its incipient stages drawing is not an entirely free assimilation of reality to the child's internal schemas because it constitutes sometimes a preparation for and sometimes a product of imitative accommodation. In this way, 'between the graphic image and the internal image (Luquet's internal model) there exist innumerable interactions, since both phenomena derive directly from imitation' (Piaget and Inhelder 1969: 63). Therefore, although children may begin by drawing what they know rather than what they see, they eventually become guided by attempts to realistically imitate phenomena. Piaget qualifies this view by referring to Luquet who proposes that visual realism in drawing passes through several developmental phases. These are worth outlining because of their widespread influence on research into children's drawing.

The first phase is *fortuitous realism*, which refers to the realism

91

children discover in their own scribble. Then appears *failed realism*, or the phase of synthetic incapacity in which the visual elements of a picture are juxtaposed instead of being coordinated into a whole. Hats are drawn apart from heads, coat buttons separate from coats, and so forth.[4] This is followed by *intellectual realism*, when drawing has evolved beyond primitive scribblings but where it depicts the conceptual attributes of the model without concern for perspective. A face in profile is portrayed as having two eyes (because children *know* faces possess two eyes); trees are seen 'through' normally occluding houses (transparency), and so forth. The last of Luquet's stages is *visual realism*, when two new features are introduced into children's drawing. First, they represent what is visible from one perspective; second, concealed parts of the object are no longer represented. At this final stage, then, children concentrate on representing the purely visual aspects of the world as seen from a fixed perspective (cf. Luquet 1913, 1927).

In summary, then, Piaget argues that children's development is strongly influenced by intersensorial perception which involves complex sensori-motor activitity. This argument strongly contributes to his views on children's drawing in that, such is the nature of children's genetic development in the light of experience, the visual world is not conceived of in isolation but has meaning only as a part of a total universe. (These views provide a developmental basis for those of Dreyfus, reviewed in chapter 4, that our higher cognitions are only possible because of our status as sensory beings. It is this *embodied* condition that allows information to be shared among our sensory systems and it is our capacity to correlate this information that lends it significance.)[5]

5.3 THE HOLISTIC NATURE OF CHILDREN'S DRAWING

Piaget's view that visual perception has meaning only as a part of a total universe strengthens my own that pictures can elicit memory traces of our intersensorially mediated understanding of phenomena. It also suggests that when children reach the stage of graphically representing their understanding of the unfolding world, they do not concentrate on its purely visual aspects. That is, if children's evolved and lived understanding of the world is intersensorially mediated, these relations surely affect their intentions toward specific subjects, including those they attempt to represent in their drawing. This contention is schematized in 5.

Schema 5

phenomenal world → intersensorially mediated experience of
world affects children's understanding of and intentions
toward → phenomenal world represented in drawing.

I am proposing that – *just as pictures elicit from us more than our
visually encapsulated knowledge of the world, children attempt to project
into their drawing such non-visually derived knowledge*. Children's drawing should therefore be approached as a complex act and not solely
in terms of attempts to find structural equivalents for their exclusively visually perceived understanding of the world. Approached
as an holistic act, drawing can be seen as offering children a relatively direct and intuitive means of communicating what I describe
as their *holistic mental intentions*. In this way, drawing does not offer
children merely a passive 'camera-like' means of recording their
visual perceptions of phenomena.

I also think it true that children's holistic intentions toward drawing can typically result in confusion from the point of view of visual
realism. In Piagetian terms, it can be said that, because children
are concerned with communicating their 'heterogeneous schemata' in their drawing, they fail to properly single out, for the
purposes of visually representing the world in two dimensions, the
elements that exclusively constitute their visual schemata. Therefore, although it might be that things visual have meaning only as
a part of a total universe, children initially do not realize that, by
and large, this universe in all its diversity cannot be adequately
visually communicated. Regardless, therefore, they begin by
attempting to visually represent their heterogeneous but *undifferentiated* schemata in their drawing or else in the behaviour that
accompanies it. From this it follows that, although the material results of the drawing act appear to be confined to the visual, what
can be thought of as children's *visually embodied intention*, this is
necessarily so because of the material constraints inherent in the
drawing medium (pencils, crayons, paper, etc.).

As they mature, however, children become increasingly cognizant of the communicative constraints inherent in the drawing
medium and this results in their developing a symbol system capable of objectively representing the purely visual properties of a

subject from a fixed perspective. This process leads to a marked improvement in children's drawing from the point of view of visual realism. Luquet's developmental stages can therefore be partially explained in terms of children's increasing capacity to differentiate the nature of their perceptions for the purposes of objectively representing visual reality in two dimensions.[6]

Nonetheless, although it may be that children's drawing becomes progressively realistic, it seems to me that we can learn a great deal about the complex nature of adult picture perception by examining children's drawing prior to the visual realism phase. My proposal is that certain belief systems that manifest themselves in an *overt* form as a part of children's drawing, remain covertly mentally active in adulthood to affect picture perception. By attempting to understand how children *draw*, therefore, we should be able to gain cognitive insights into how we *see*.

5.4 THE HIDDEN MEANING IN CHILDREN'S DRAWING

If, because of intersensorial perception, children's drawing is holistically mentally intentioned, we should expect to find some evidence of this either in the drawing itself or else in the behaviour that accompanies it. In fact, we find both behavioural and visual evidence that children are influenced by more than their exclusively visually derived perceptions of the world.

Korzenik, in her study on how children come to *decontextualize* themselves from their drawing, observed their behaviour before this process occurs.[7] In one example she tells us how Billy patted his stomach after a big supper while saying, 'Here's where my ice-cream is'. He subsequently grasped a crayon, swung a full circle shape in the air and then drew a circular mark accompanied by, 'See, I'm big and full'. He then formed a mark inside the circle accompanied by, 'Here's where the ice-cream's melting' (1977: 192).

It is pointed out that, because Billy's overt behaviour occurred outside the graphic medium of crayon and paper, only an observer present at the time would have known all the things Billy represented to himself. A true understanding of his picture would therefore be impossible for someone absent from the context in which it was made. Korzenik therefore concludes that children's drawing is not, as is sometimes supposed, a case of merely photographically replicating the world, and she continues:

> This misconception pervades much of the research on child-
> ren's drawings; it can perhaps be attributed to the habit of
> analysing pictures in isolation, apart from the child and from
> the problem he attempted to solve. To correct this, not only
> the final product but also its accompanying observable behav-
> iour must be assessed.
>
> (Korzenik 1977: 192)

After presenting us with further examples of children's behaviour when drawing, Korzenik proposes that as they become
increasingly less egocentric they become aware that pictures cannot
depend for their intelligibility upon a context outside the graphic
medium. This realization leads children to increasingly decontextualize themselves from their drawing and results in a tendency
towards visual realism.

Eng points out that, when drawing, children often imagine they
are performing certain actions which, in addition to their visual
output, is described in both words and gestures. We are told how
four-year-old Gunter wished to represent 'on' his drawing by 'clos-
ing a curtain', that night had arrived. He energetically passed his
pencil from top to bottom over his paper as if pulling a curtain
cord. No misunderstanding was possible, says Eng, 'It was not the
cord itself, but the action of drawing it, which was to be expressed by the motion of the drawing pencil in a similar direction'
(1966: 171).

Both Korzenik and Eng's observations are confirmed by my own.
I recall the behaviour displayed by one child when representing
'battling fighter jets'. After drawing several jets spread over the
paper he subsequently began to introduce some 'action' into the
scene. This was visually communicated by a series of short 'staccato'
lines meant as equivalents for the trajectories of the jets' rockets
in motion. The paper quickly became replete with criss-crossing
lines, some of these finding their 'target' (other jets), others 'missing' and trailing off into 'space' (the edges of the paper). The
child's face was stern and concentrated as he drew these lines and
when he engineered one to 'make a hit' this was typically accompanied by an appropriately orally produced 'exploding' sound and
a frenetic scribble on the paper where the 'hit' was made. The child
was clearly living out, moment by moment, his holistic, intersen-

sorially mediated comprehension of the scene, when appropriate using his body as a symbolic vehicle. This would have been impossible to discern by looking at the child's visually embodied intention, the drawing itself. Its criss-crossing lines in fact eventually resulted in visual confusion.

There is often strong visual evidence in children's drawing indicating the influence of their general understanding of a subject. Eng observes that when children draw houses, for example, they are gradually 'fitted out' in increasing detail – staircases, tiles on the roof and curtains are added. It is further pointed out:

> Very often we are allowed a view of the interior of the house, we see tables, chairs and other necessary objects which the child supposes to exist in every house, and hence must also be drawn; furthermore, the inhabitants of the house appear, they stand up next to their house, or they are seated inside at table.
>
> (Eng 1966: 122)

Eng continues by noting that children first usually draw a house from one side only, but because they know it has several sides, they often make some attempt to draw these too. After the acquisition of some elementary visual knowledge, however, they draw only the sides that they can actually see and often attempt a true perspectival representation. And Eng proposes in general, 'The house is an early and favourite model for the child, because it is interested in it and has a well-formed mental picture.' (122–3). Regarding the child's mental picture (or mental image, as it is currently known), Eng suggests:

> The free drawing of children before the school age is almost entirely from memory, and for the most part it remains the same during the early years at school. Children do not look at the things that they wish to represent, but draw them out of their heads from their mental picture of them.
>
> (Eng 1966: 124)

Goodnow also implies that children's drawing is holistically intentioned when she proposes that one aspect of working with shapes has to do with how we learn how one thing (one shape) can stand for something else, but the two can mean the same thing. Learning *equivalence* in this way is a constant part of our lives occurring each time we apply with precision the terms 'same' and 'different'. We are asked to consider some of the more obvious equivalents used in drawing. The shape of the mouth (up, down or straight) stands for various feelings. The position of pupils in the eyes (centre, side, top) stand for the direction of the gaze. The bottom part of the page stands for ground, the top for the sky, hair flying stands for the effects of wind or running, and so forth (1977: 112). And it is argued in general that:

> A short check list on comic-strips and book illustrations will yield many more equivalents ... and it will also yield with a sense of surprise that so many equivalents exist for feeling, position, time, sound movement, collision, intention, and so on, even in work intended to be easily interpreted by children.
>
> (Goodnow 1977: 112)

Goodnow's views might be put differently by saying that pictures are often replete with equivalents for our intersensorially mediated understanding of the world and they are therefore about more than our purely visual understanding of the world as we perceive it reduced to two dimensions. In conclusion, Goodnow proposes that children's graphic work illustrates our thinking as well as theirs:

> Graphic work is truly 'visible thinking'. The features it displays – thrift, conservatism, principles of organization and sequence – are features of all problem solving, whether by children or adults. If you begin to note these features in one area of experience – children's graphic work – then you may begin to note them in your own thinking and problem solving.
>
> (Goodnow 1977: 154)

Korzenik reaches similar conclusions when, regarding her question: What happens then to all that is no longer compatible with the adult's use of pictorial communication? – she answers:

> They may yet be retained in the mind for private fantasy and logical problem solving. Private visual thinking may enable a person to address a problem in ways that are visual and yet beyond the pragmatic limits of the graphic medium's capability.
>
> (Korzenik 1977: 206)

These views complement my own that certain belief systems manifested in some explicit form as a part of children's drawing, remain 'covertly' active in adulthood to affect picture perception.

I shall conclude this section by concentrating on an important aspect of children's figure drawing, the human head. It is well established that an overwhelming tendency exists to draw the head larger than the trunk well into middle childhood, as Eng notes, 'The commonest mistake in the child's representation of the human figure is that of making the head too large' (1966: 162). It is proposed that this 'mistake' could be that children emphasize in their drawing what appears interesting or important, frequently making it disproportionately large.

Freeman comments similarly that children's tendency to visually exaggerate head size could be an example of 'a photographically erroneous advance planning whereby relative size is used as a convention to signal relative importance' (1980: 228).

Selfe also remarks on children's tendency to overestimate head size and comments that, 'There are surprisingly few studies of the development of photographically realistic proportions in human figure drawing' (1983: 48).

Selfe attempted to remedy this situation by testing the assumption that the human figure body-part proportions show developmental sensitivity in the direction of more photographically realistic productions with age (thereby substantiating Luquet's model reviewed earlier). Results of the tests showed that on average, 5–6 year-olds draw the head larger than the trunk. By 7–8 years, the child draws the trunk slightly larger than the head size, and by 9–10, it produces a trunk approximately three times larger than the head size. From these results Selfe concludes, 'Even by the age of ten years then, the normal child has some way to go before representing photographically realistic proportions in their human figure drawing' (49).

Finally, it is worth noting Eng's comments on pictorial representation of the head itself. She points out that it is generally shown as a circle, sometimes as an oval but rarely as a rectangle. Regarding the importance of facial features, eyes are drawn in first and rarely forgotten; they are often drawn as points, circles, points surrounded by circles and, as children develop, eyebrows are shown by curved lines. Although the mouth is sometimes forgotten, it is the next most important feature and often represented by a line crossing the whole of the face, as two parallel lines, as an oval and may sometimes be rectangularly or spindle-shaped. The nose is frequently omitted because in full-face it is not obviously significant (as it might be in profile). When drawn, it is represented as a circle, straight line, oval, triangle, rectangle, or crooked line. The ears are usually drawn as rounded figures standing out from each side of the head, and in profile they are represented as ovals (Eng 1966: 112–13)

I have been able to no more than briefly review selected aspects of research on children's drawing, a vast and still relatively uncharted area in its own right. The studies I have referred to are therefore not necessarily representative of the researchers' major themes. Nonetheless, I shall now attempt to show that their insights into children's drawing are relevant to adult picture perception.

5.5 THE LINK BETWEEN CHILDREN'S DRAWING AND ADULT PICTURE PERCEPTION

By drawing attention to the observation that children's drawings of houses often include interiors, Eng substantiates Luquet's *intellectual realism* phase when drawing depicts the conceptual aspects of the model without perspectival concerns.[8] The adult representational artist, however, whose work conforms to the rules associated with visual realism, is conscious that when representing a scene from a fixed perspective some of the objects represented will occlude others, as in reality. A house will be represented with the outside walls occluding its interior, although parts may be shown 'through' a window or open door. From the point of view of realism this is acceptable simply because standing in front of a house we often do see aspects of its interior through windows and open doors. Similarly, if representing an interior including a window, it is quite acceptable to include an 'outside' view as seen 'through' the window, and so forth.

Nonetheless, the child's apparently confused and naive drawing informs us more about the 'hidden' nature of our perceptions than does the sophisticated representation. On perceiving a visually realistic image of a house we intuitively assume than an interior 'exists' behind its façade – we do not typically believe that we are perceiving a two-dimensional film prop, for example. This is the case paradoxically, in spite of the fact that, on one level of con-

99

sciousness, we are aware that the representation is a mere illusion because of its two dimensionality. And here, I am not talking about *trompe-l'œil*, which sets out to confuse realities, but ordinary pictures that are fully accepted as illusions. Similarly, on perceiving a picture of even a part of a room, we tend to assume its complete existential identity as a part of a house – we do not assume that the part we see is all that exists.

In children's drawing, however, the experiential component is not merely implied (the interior 'behind' the house façade, etc.) but explicitly represented in the drawing itself. Children are therefore communicating: We *know* that houses have interiors, often full of interesting things, as you can *see*. This complements my view of adult picture perception which goes something like: We know that houses have interiors, *in spite of what we see*.

The tendency towards transparency is not confined to children, however. Eng points out that in Giotto's *The Pope's Dream* in the Monastery Church at Assisi, and in *Zacharias in the Temple* in Santa Croce in Florence, the artist represents a house from the front and makes its walls transparent so that the life and action of the people inside can be seen. (1966: 124). Many like examples can be found in the history of art.

Also significant about children's tendency towards transparency, which is typically executed without reference to the model, is that it helps to substantiate Piaget's view of the mental image – of it being an *active* copy of perceptual data consequent upon participation in events. That is, in order for children to represent a multi-dimensional view of a house, they surely have to draw from complex but internally coherent representations constructed from life experience. Further, this experience will surely include certain sensori-motor related activities such as walking from the outside to the inside of houses, up stairs, and so forth.

From a neuropsychological perspective, this hypothetical relationship between sensory motor activity, sensorily perceived information and the mental image, shares aspects in common with my own views and perhaps those of Springer and Deutsch referred to in chapter 3. For example, their view that areas of the right hemisphere evolved ways of presenting abstractly two- and three-dimensional relationships of the external world grasped through vision, touch and movement. (There is increasing evidence that mental imagery is a primarily, although not exclusively, right-hemisphere associated phenomenon. See Ley 1982.)

If children's drawings of houses can inform us about adult picture perception, then so too can their tendency to exaggerate head size in figure drawing. As with transparency, this perception is not alien to the history of art. In Giotto's *Ognissanti Madonna*, the central figures of mother and child tower over their attendant angels leaving us in no doubt as to who are the protagonists of the scene. This accentuation is not only communicated through the diminutive angels but also through the direction of their (adulatory) gaze.

The head and face do not have to be visually exaggerated to capture our attention. When represented in perfect proportion to the rest of the body we still tend to concentrate on their form and meaning. For example, our perceptions of Holbein's *Georg Gisze* are immediately drawn to the head of the figure and particularly to the eyes which dominate the picture (Figure 7). We experience no difficulty in interpreting the expression on the face although it exhibits no strong emotion. And yet the face is by no means the only image in the picture competing for our attention: we also find flowers, books, shelves, papers, and so forth. Although it may be that we are eventually drawn to these and they constitute an important part of the picture perceived as a whole, we are continually drawn back to the face and eyes.

It seems to me that the reason our perception of *Georg Gisze* is controlled in this way strongly relates to why it is children visually exaggerate heads in their drawing. That is, as the single most communicative part of the human anatomy, the head is valued above all other parts.[9] Consequently, whereas the importance of the head is overtly visually stated in children's drawing, in more visually accomplished pictures its meaning remains visually 'hidden' – but its effect no less powerful. And here it is worth reminding ourselves that facial recognition is overwhelmingly associated with right-hemisphere function (Hecaen and Angelergues 1962; Levy *et al.* 1972, for example).

There are further aspects of children's drawing that can tell us about our perceptions of *Georg Gisze* and by implication other visual representations. As indicated by Goodnow (1977), children quickly come to think of the bottom half of the paper as the 'ground', the top half as the 'sky'. Within this conceptual space, torsoes' axes are usually drawn vertical for a standing figure, the head placed above the torso, the legs beneath, 'touching the ground' and so forth, as

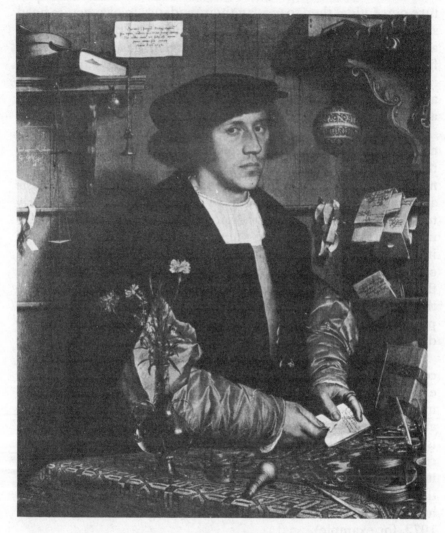

Figure 7 Hans Holbein (1497–1543) *Georg Gisze*, wood, 96 × 85.7 cm
Source: Staatliche Museum, Berlin

in real life. In addition to showing that children develop a sense of visual proportion this indicates their intuitive grasp of the effects of gravity, as do the results of Goodnow's request that children should draw someone picking up a ball. In most instances it was simply assumed that the ball was positioned on the 'ground' with the implication that children's experientially derived knowledge informed them that, by and large, stationary balls are gravitationally bound. Goodnow's request complements my own when I asked children to draw scenes from a local fair. These often included balloons which, although also drawn ball-like, were automatically positioned 'floating' well above the ground line.

From this it follows that one of the ways in which children learn how one thing (one shape) can stand for something else, is by contextualizing it in the light of their intersensorially mediated understanding of the shape's phenomenal referent, stored in memory.[10]

Not only can we observe the sky/ground equivalent in *Georg Gisze* but also equivalents for the effects of gravity; the central figure and all other objects in the picture conform to its laws. The scales to the left of the picture, 'suspended' in mid-space, 'resist' gravity only because of their suspension by a cord, as is true of the ball to the right of the figure. The books and boxes above the scales and ball fail to topple over because they are 'supported' by shelves; the objects 'placed' on the table conform to the same gravitational laws, and so forth.

What is relevant about these observations is the clear implication that we intuitively apply our general, intersensorially mediated understanding of an image's phenomenal referents to the image itself regardless of our better knowledge that it is mere illusion. Put differently, such is the nature of our development that, in Piagetian terms, we have assimilated scales, books, boxes, etc. to the separate schemata of weighing, friction, falling, and so forth, and accordingly apply this understanding to pictures. Experience informs us that the density of certain visually identifiable objects is such that they are incapable of existing in space without support – and we find it strange if they are represented in a picture as having no support, as is often the case in the work of René Magritte.

I have, then, proposed that we quite intuitively transfer many of the structures developed in childhood and associated with life values, to pictures with the implication that picture perception is about more than responding to the purely visual. This is by no means agreed, however, as we shall see in the next chapter when I review certain theories of picture perception. I shall conclude this chapter, however, by speculating on the role cerebral lateralization of function plays in children's drawing.

5.6   LATERALIZATION OF FUNCTION AND CHILDREN'S DRAWING

One of the difficulties involved in rigorously applying insights gained from lateralization research to children is that they possess a greater potential for cerebral plasticity of function than do adults, as we saw in chapter 3. We also saw in this chapter that it is still uncertain at what stage in child development the corpus callosum becomes fully myelinated and therefore functional, that is, capable of exchanging in some form initially primarily unilaterally registered information. In addition, children are insufficiently mentally developed to be capable of even attempting to linguistically account for their behaviour. What these factors amount to is that it is difficult to attribute with any certainty specific activities as being dominantly lateralized in the still-developing child.

This notwithstanding, my view is that because of the relations between drawing and the phenomenal world, it offers children a relatively direct, intuitive and non-discursively associated means of coming to terms with their unfolding awareness. Given what I have argued from a neuropsychological perspective, from this it follows that drawing is a dominantly right-hemisphere activity in the child.

This view shares aspects in common with those of Gazzaniga on mental organization as reviewed in chapter 4, and which he confirms elsewhere:

> My interpretation is that the normal brain is organized into modular processing systems ... and that these modules can usually express themselves only through real action, not through verbal communication. Most of these systems ... can remember events, store affective reactions to those events, and respond to stimuli associated with a particular memory.
> (Gazzaniga 1985: 77)

Given that drawing constitutes a form of real action, therefore, it can be seen as offering the child a relatively direct means of responding to its intersensorially mediated memory understanding of the world.

Although it may be the case that drawing is a dominantly right-hemisphere associated activity, there are clear signs that it can involve linguistic or quasi-linguistic associated strategies. This is first evidenced by the fact that children often accompany their drawing with verbal statements. Billy accompanied his drawing of himself as being 'big and full' with a verbal statement to that effect. This is relevant because the strategies underlying such accompaniments perhaps share aspects in common with the phylogenetic emergence of lateralization as argued in chapter 3. Regarding the Neanderthal, for example, the capacity to gesturally denote a snake by an undulatory motion of the arm or hand, implies the use of both iconic and arbitrary classes of symbol-forming. That is, the motion may have served as a quasi-iconic reminder of man's visual understanding of snakes' movement patterns and also been capable of denoting something about the class of species, thereby implying the capacity to name and classify things in the world.

Luquet's *failed realism* drawing phase also indicates the intervention of a drawing strategy associated with language. That is, hats drawn above and buttons apart from bodies implies the use of a linguistically associated 'listing' strategy.[11] (This strategy could share aspects in common with the one that led the Neanderthal to carve into iconic artifacts sequentially oriented marks symptomatic of a proto-language, as reviewed in chapter 3.)

It is not necessarily the case, however, that the intervention of linguistically associated strategies enhances children's potential to successfully visually communicate their evolving understanding of the world. Children's attempts to 'list' the characteristics of an object without proper concern for placement is no more visually successful than would be an attempt to communicate a linguistic message without conforming to the rules of syntax. A linguistic message as communicated in schema 6 is incomprehensible.

Schema 6

is	upon	wearing	he	coat	a	
head	and	also	his	wearing		
man	this	hat	a	is	buttons	with

However, if presented in accordance with syntactical rules, the message makes good sense: This man is wearing a hat upon his head and he is also wearing a coat with buttons.

In fact, Selfe (1977, 1983, 1985) concludes from her research on a selected group of autistic children that their serious difficulties with language acquisition enhanced their potential to draw visually realistic pictures. She argues that without linguistic dominance and

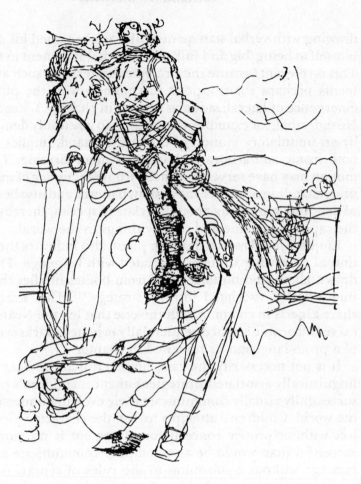

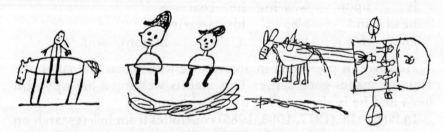

Figure 8   Drawing of a horse by Nadia, aged 5, compared to drawings
of children of a comparative age

Source: Selfe 1977

mediation in early years of development, when graphic competence was being acquired, the children were able to concentrate on the spatial characteristic of their optic array and this was reflected in their drawing: 'These children ... have a more direct access to visual imagery in the sense that their drawings are not so strongly "contaminated" by the usual "designating and naming" properties of normal children's drawings' (1983: 201).

Certainly the drawings of the autistic child Nadia are exceptional and particularly when contrasted with drawings done by normal children of a similar or older age (Figure 8). It should be noted, however, that in addition to her linguistic incompetence, Nadia was never seen to indulge in symbolic play and that her gross motor development was poor: she could neither hop nor walk up stairs one at a time, for example.

Given Piaget's account of the mental image as being an *active* copy of perceptual data consequent upon events beings participated in by the child, it could follow that not only Nadia's linguistic abilities but also her mental imagery potential remained underdeveloped. Further, given Piaget's account of drawing as lying somewhere between symbolic play and the mental image, it could be that the lack of these competences in Nadia, along with her linguistic inadequacy, affected her drawing abilities. (Selfe might not agree with this, however. See Selfe 1983: 13–14).

Nonetheless, language clearly can play some part in mediating children's drawing even if this mediation only adds to the drawing's confusion. It could be, then, that in children's drawing the two distinct symbol forms related to language and image-making sometimes 'compete' for the right to symbolically output information. This is perhaps because, from a neuropsychological perspective, the mental systems associated with these distinct symbol forms have not yet become sufficiently 'hardwired' in the child's still developing brain. This has the effect that the cognitive strategies associated with language- and image-making more readily mutually interfere than at later stages of cognitive development.

With a cognitive maturation of the brain, however, these systems become increasingly cerebrally localized and independent with the result that the older child becomes more readily capable of differentiating the qualitative and communicative constraints inherent in distinct classes of symbol-forming. That is, the child comes to realize that successful visual communication does not necessarily imply successful linguistic communication, and vice versa. This view agrees with the one I hypothesized regarding our phylogeny. That is, the left hemisphere's increasing preoccupation with language functions facilitated the right hemisphere's potential to develop unique non-linguistic capacities of an iconic and phenomenally related class.

5.7 SUMMARY

Piaget's contention that visual perception has meaning only as a part of ar 'ntersensorially mediated 'total universe' strengthens my own that pictures elicit more than their visually encapsulated knowledge of phenomena. If from an early age children's drawing is intersensorially mediated and holistically mentally intentioned, we should expect to find evidence of this in their drawing or in the behaviour that accompanies it. By looking at these signs we should discover something about adult picture perception.

Transparency in children's drawing informs us about how we intuitively contextualize two-dimensional representations of three-dimensional objects by referring to our experientially derived understanding of their referents. Their tendency to overestimate head size indicates why it might be that our attentions are drawn to realistically proportioned pictures of heads. Their intuitive use of the top and bottom of drawing paper as equivalents for sky and ground, coupled with how objects are positioned within this conceptual space, further informs us about our perceptual assumptions. For example, that objects are associated with particular functions; that they possess certain densities and weights; that they are affected by gravitational laws. In general, then, children's drawing explicitly indicates that we intuitively transfer many of the structures associated with life values to pictures of the world. Finally, children's drawing is a dominantly but not exclusively right-hemisphere associated activity.

Chapter Six

THE LANGUAGES OF ART

6.1 INTRODUCTION

Drawing from the neuropsychological evidence, I have concluded that picture perception is a complex holistic mental process involving reference primarily to our right-hemisphere associated, non-discursive but intersensorially mediated experience of phenomena. This view brings me to the 'translation issue' referred to in the introduction and centring around the question of the extent to which language can plausibly explicate the representational visual image. In this chapter I pursue the argument that the extent is limited because the two symbol systems involved are constructed from and elicit different ways of knowing or processing information.

I shall begin by saying something about theories of picture perception, however, because certain of these argue that we learn to see pictures in something like the same way that we learn to read writing or acquire a language. This has the implication that pictures bear no intrinsic relation to their referents thereby supporting the argument that they benefit from linguistically formulated explanations – in the same way that the meaning of a foreign language benefits by being translated into our native tongue. If pictures are understood in virtue of their iconicity, however, this goes some way to weakening this argument. That is, if they automatically trigger our visual and more general life understanding of their referents, it surely follows that this understanding plays the major part in determining their meaning.

6.2   DO WE LEARN TO SEE PICTURES?

Kennedy argues that theories of picture perception can be summarized as variations on four major themes.

> Pictures are simply conventions, no more related to what
> they represent than alphabetic writing; second, that pictures
> are simply similar to what they depict; third, that pictures
> provide the same elements of light as represented objects or
> scenes; fourth, that pictures provide the same optic informa-
> tion as the pictured objects or scenes.
>
> (Kennedy 1974: 29)

The last three themes each imply in their way that the capacity to make sense of pictures is innate, or at least as innately determined as the one we habitually employ to understand the visual nature of objects in the world. The first theory, often described as the *conventional* theory, suggests that pictures bear no intrinsic relation to what they represent with the implication that their meaning depends upon some form of social convention that has to be learned.[1]

The conventional theory is advanced by Steinberg (1953) when he proposes that the purported visual skill to imitate nature is a fallacy; rather, what is developed is the skill of reproducing graphic symbols by set professional conventions. Although less strong, Arnheim implies similar conclusions when he argues:

> We must go further and realize that just as persons of our
> own civilization and century may perceive a particular man-
> ner of representation as lifelike even though it may not look
> lifelike at all to adherents of another approach, so do the ad-
> herents of those other approaches find their preferred man-
> ner of representation not only acceptable, but entirely
> lifelike.[2]
>
> (Arnheim 1974: 136)

This view that visual realism in pictures is not universally perceptible echoes Goodman's theme when he says, 'Realism is relative, determined by the system of representation standard for a given culture or person at a given time. Newer or older or alien systems are accounted artificial or unskilled' (1968: 37). Goodman, however, is best known for his conclusion that, 'Realistic representation ... depends not upon imitation or illusion or information but upon inculcation. Almost any picture may represent almost anything; that is, given picture and object there is usually a system of representation, a plan or correlation, under which the picture represents the object. How correct the picture is under that system depends upon how accurate is the information about the object that is obtained by reading the picture according to that system.' (1968: 38).

Although at a first reading this conclusion is certainly provocative, the point that there is usually a plan or correlation under which the picture represents the object in fact amounts to no more than a truism. Clearly such a correlation exists – given that, by definition, a picture cannot in material terms be the object it *re*presents. The important issue is whether this correlation is sufficiently optically similar to its referent to be recognized without formal learning or whether it is arbitrary and needs to be learned. Goodman's argument that any picture can represent almost anything clearly suggests that he favours the latter view, as he confirms elsewhere, 'how literal or realistic the picture is depends on how standard the system is. If representation is a matter of choice and correctness a matter of information, realism is a matter of habit' (1968: 38).

Eco also implies that pictures are constructed from conventions when he proposes that we succeed in understanding a given technical solution as a representation of a natural experience because there has been informed in us a codified system of expectations which allow us to enter the semantic world of the artist. In this way:

> Maybe an 'iconic' solution is not conventional when it is proposed, but it becomes so step by step, the more its addressee becomes acquainted with it. At a certain point the iconic representation, however stylized it may be, appears to be more true than the real experience, and people begin to look at things through the glasses of iconic convention.
>
> (Eco 1976: 204–5)

Eco states elsewhere:

> But the real puzzling problem is not so much how one may represent a man with ten eyes and seven legs as why one may *visually represent (and recognize as represented)* a given man with

111

two eyes and *two* legs. How is it possible to represent a man standing and a lady sitting under a tree, a calm landscape with clouds and a corn-field behind them, a given light and a given mood – as happens in Gainsborough's *Mr and Mrs Andrews*?

(Eco 1976: 249–250)

Eco fails to realize, however, as do proponents of the conventional theory in general, although it is true that we are unlikely to have experienced exactly the same visual elements as those constituting *Mr and Mrs Andrews*, the reason we have little difficulty in recognizing its forms is because they *sufficiently* accord with our optical experience of the phenomenal world, that is, what human beings, dogs, trees, and clouds actually *look like*. If this initial relation were not paramount it would be difficult to explain how we comprehend Gainsborough's stylistic inclination to elongate his figures, given that elongation implies a prior knowledge of the typical size of an object. As we have seen, Eco would probably disagree, because, 'At a certain point, the iconic representation, however stylized it may be, appears to be more real than the real experience'. This has the implication that Gainsborough's elongated figures come to be perceived as more 'real' than an averagely proportioned figure. (The corollary assumption being that, after having become sufficiently acquainted with Gainsborough's tendency to elongate we subsequently perceive averagely proportioned figures in everyday life as stunted.)

This is not to pretend that style plays no part in picture perception or that we might not take longer to familiarize ourselves with certain styles than others. As Gombrich (1977) discusses at length, Constable's public initially found his (then contemporary) work difficult to assimilate whereas now it instigates no such difficulties, etc. Nonetheless, whereas Gombrich admits to some of Eco's views on the nature of *similitude* (it is produced and must be learned), he makes the point that:

Western art would not have developed the special tricks of naturalism if it had not found that the incorporation in the image of all the features which serve us in real life for the discovery and testing of meaning enabled the artist to do with fewer and fewer conventions.

(Gombrich 1982: 287)[3]

Gombrich substantiates this view elsewhere when he argues that it seems unlikely that the responses to the 'erotic nudes' displayed on the covers and pages of magazines on sale in our cities depends upon 'inculcation', so that, 'To be sure, there are conventions at work in the choice of the models and of the poses, but the aim must be to produce the maximum permitted effect' (1982: 297). The implication is that visual erotica of the class found in *Playboy* is not only instantly recognizable but also capable of producing a definite response when perceived in terms of its referents. Therefore, although a percipient may be aware that a picture of a woman in a sexually clichéd pose has something of the iconic convention about it, prior to this awareness there surely exists a biologically involved tendency to relate to the naked female form – and does not a similar principle play its part in our relations to Boucher's *Reclining Girl* (Figure 9), in spite of its assured place in the history of art?[4]

To underline the view that, by and large, pictures are understood in virtue of their iconicity, I paged through Gombrich's *The Story of Art* (1967 version) which includes over 380 illustrations whose referents date from 30,000 BC to the present century. The purpose of this exercise was to see how many of the illustrations were not immediately recognizable as bearing some relation to their referents. There were only ten even when the information provided was only minimal. I thus experienced no difficulty in recognizing cave drawings of a bison and reindeer produced in 15,000 BC. This surely goes a long way to proving the universal and time-transcending communicative power of representational imagery – given that the cave dwellers of Altamira and Fonte de Gaume lived remarkably different cultural lives from our own.

Further and more conclusive evidence that picture perception is an innately determined ability comes from a seminal experiment conducted by Hochberg and Brooks (1962). The researchers raised their child with restricted exposure to any kind of picture. Labels were removed from cans and bottles and no picture books were allowed so that the child had minimal practice in seeing the meanings and spatial relations in two-dimensional representations and designs. Also, the child was never instructed in associations between words or pictures, or told that pictures represent anything, and he was never read a story accompanied by illustrations.

Just before the child was 20 years old, by which time it had a reasonably large vocabulary, it was shown line drawings and monochromatic photographs of objects and asked what they represented.

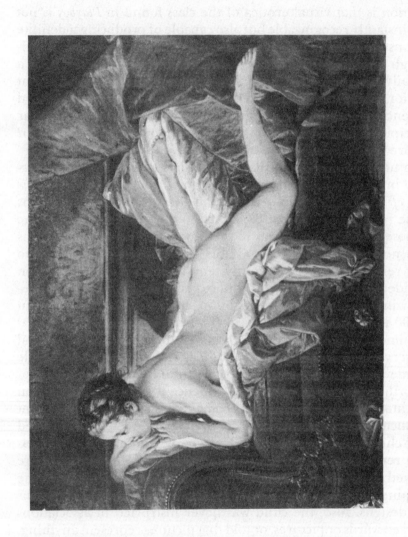

Figure 9 François Boucher (1703–1770) *Reclining Girl*, canvas 59 × 73 cm

Source: Alte Pinakothek, Munich

Almost all of the pictures were correctly labelled regardless of whether they were photographs, complex line drawings with interior detail, or simply outline drawings with only one interior line. From this result it was reasonably concluded that our capacity to understand pictures is innately determined and not reliant upon any form of social learning.

The view that pictures are understood in virtue of their iconicity has been developed by Kennedy (1974), particularly regarding outline drawings. He argues that anything in the phenomenal world that has distinctive features of shape and is visible should be identifiable in outline because, 'The power of outlines does not rest on showing whole objects, which of course they can do, but on being able to present information for the fundamental features of the visible environment' (132). And he continues:

> Outline drawings capitalize on ecological information provided by distinctive features of shape and permit observers without training or captions to identify basic discontinuities of shape, slant, pigment, illumination and texture. Outline can depict discontinuities without reproducing the colors or textures or intensities that define each discontinuity, by presenting the informative variables of shapes that help distinguish each discontinuity.
>
> (Kennedy 1974: 133)

This argument that we recognize outline drawings because they capitalize on ecological information clearly complements Marr's emphasis that our visual system developed as a result of our goal-oriented needs as a species, as reviewed in chapter 3. Thus, even stick figures of mammals constructed from pipe cleaners, although offering minimal visual information, make sense to us because they resemble the lines the brain in fact computes.

(In fact, if we consider the diverse ways in which pictures are capable of communicating the visual nature of their referent forms, this suggests the following possibility. It could be that when presented with visual marks that correspond to perhaps only one of Marr's 'computational stages' (the primal sketch, the 2½-D sketch, etc.) these are sufficient to trigger the remaining stages thereby affording a picture its complete 3-D model identity from minimal information. This would help to explain how we recognize pictures when they fail to visually match their referents in all re-

115

spects, which is usually the case. It would also help to explain how, contra to the conventional theory, many pictures from different cultures, although perhaps emphasizing different classes of visual information (outline, shading, etc.), are universally recognizable without training in their conventions. The possibility is that pictures do not need to visually correspond in all respects to their referents because, such is the evolved nature of our visual system, we automatically 'compute' the parts not shown.)[5]

In conclusion, then, if pictures are understood in virtue of their iconicity, as I have argued, this goes some way to weakening the argument that they require some form of linguistically formulated knowledge for their explanation. That is, if pictures trigger our visual and, by implication, our more general life understanding of their referents, it surely follows that this understanding plays the major part in determining their meaning.

6.3 ART AS LITERATURE?

In this section I introduce Panofsky's views because, while they indicate that certain representational images are understood as containing life values, this (direct) perception is considered undesirable unless qualified by forms of literary knowledge.

Panofsky (1955) argues that our 'correct' response to certain works of representational visual art should be guided by three levels of description. The most basic level is *pre-iconographical description* which relates to identifying pure forms. That is, certain configurations of line and colour or certain lumps of bronze or stone, are identified as representing natural objects such as human beings, animals, plants, and so forth. (In this way, Panofsky acknowledges that representational imagery is perceived in virtue of its iconicity.) These forms and their mutual relations in turn suggest expressional qualities such as the mournful character of a pose or gesture, or the homelike and peaceful atmosphere of an interior and in this way, 'The world of pure forms thus recognized as carriers of primary or natural meanings may be called the world of artistic motifs. An enumeration of these motifs would be a pre-iconographical description of the work of art' (1955: 28).

Pre-iconographical description is therefore integrally bound to how we respond to pictures in the light of our practical experience of their referents with the implication that they are about more than their purely visually encapsulated meaning.

The second level is *iconographical analysis* and concerned with connecting artistic motifs with themes or concepts. Motifs recognized as carriers of a secondary or conventional meaning are called images, and combinations of images are called stories or allegories. It is the identification of these that Panofsky sees as constituting *iconography*, and in this way:

> Iconographical analysis, dealing with images, stories and allegories instead of with motifs, presupposes, of course, much more than that familiarity with objects and events which we acquire by practical experience. It presupposes a familiarity with specific themes or concepts as transmitted through literary sources, whether acquired by purposeful reading or by oral tradition.
>
> (Panofsky 1955: 35)

Panofsky continues by arguing that, by and large, pre-iconographical responses to works of art are not in fact possible, because:

> While we believe that we are identifying the motifs on the basis of our practical experience pure and simple, we are really reading 'what we see' according to the manner in which objects and events are expressed by forms under varying historical traditions. In doing this, we subject our practical experience to a corrective principle which may be called the history of style.
>
> (Panofsky 1955: 35)[6]

The third level is *iconological interpretation* and is concerned with ascertaining those underlying principles which reveal the basic attitude of a nation, period, a class, or a religious or philosophical persuasion, qualified by one personality and condensed into their work. In conceiving of pure forms, motifs, images, and allegories as manifestations of underlying principles, they are subsequently interpreted as 'symbolic values'. It is the discovery and interpretation of these values which is the subject of *iconology*:

> Iconology ... is a method of interpretation which arises from synthesis rather than analysis. And as the correct identification of motifs is the prerequisite of their correct iconographical analysis, so is the correct analysis of images,

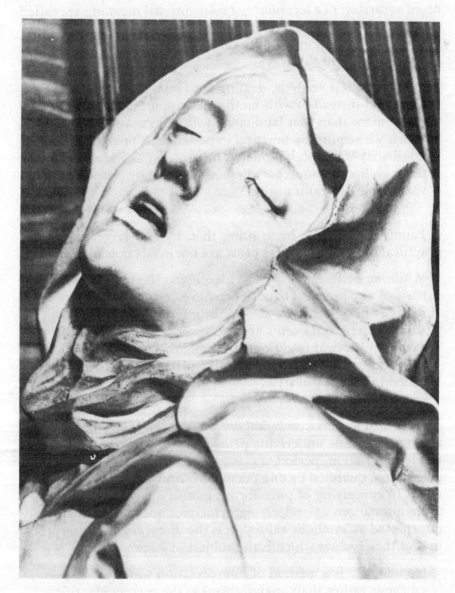

Figure 10 Gianlorenzo Bernini (1598–1680) *The Vision of Saint Theresa*
(detail), life-size figure

Source: Cornaro Chapel, S. Maria della Vittoria, Rome

stories and allegories the prerequisite of their correct iconological interpretation.

(Panofsky 1955: 32)

Panofsky illustrates iconological interpretation by applying it to
a picture of the seventeenth-century Venetian painter, Francesco
Maffei. The picture, consisting of a young woman with a sword in
her left hand and in her right a charger supporting a decapitated
head, had been published as *Salome with the Head of John the Baptist*.
It is pointed out, however, that because Salome did not personally
decapitate John, it is inconsistent that she should be holding a
sword in the picture – but it could be a portrayal of Judith who
beheaded Holofernes with her own hand. Even so, the problem
here is that the biblical text states that the head was put into a sack
and not presented on a charger. By referring to iconological interpretation, in this instance the history of types, Panofsky solves
the problem of who is being portrayed. It turns out to be Judith
because, 'while we cannot adduce a single Salome with a sword,
we encounter in Germany and North Italy, several sixteenth-cen-
tury paintings depicting Judith with a charger' (1955: 37).

In summary, then, Panofsky argues that our response to certain
works of art is essentially inadequate unless directed by specific
classes of linguistically formulated and often esoteric knowledge.
This knowledge helps constitute a major part of a hierarchically
based value system with the validity of each level of response being
qualified by the next level up within the hierarchy. In this way,
iconographical analysis involves our knowledge of concepts acquired through literary sources; iconological interpretation
requires that images, allegories, and the rest are interpreted by
broader, cross-culturally defined 'symbolic values', and so forth.

In order to fulfil all of Panofsky's conditions for the proper appreciation of certain works of art the percipient would need to be
an expert in several esoteric disciplines. It could be argued, however, that iconographical analysis is often a literary means of
distracting us from arriving at more valid conclusions, a view which
perhaps shares aspects in common with those of Pateman (1984b).

Pateman introduces his argument by putting forward a *contextualist* position, that is, one emphasizing the influence of the
cultural context in which a work of art is perceived (cf. Dickie 1974).
He continues, however, by eroding the plausibility of this position

in relation to certain art works, Bernini's *The Vision of St Theresa*, for example (Figure 10). It is one thing to see this sculpture as a woman, says Pateman, but quite another, dependent on cultural knowledge, to see it as the *Saint Theresa*, because:

> ignorant or ignoring this [religious] context of the use of the statue, you might take the expression of religious ecstasy on St Theresa's face for secular orgasm (as indeed does the French psychoanalyst Jacques Lacan: 'She's coming. No doubt about it' he says). In other words, the contextualist can now say: even something as apparently natural and non-textual as facial expression is, in fact, not independent of large scale context, the context of use.
>
> (Pateman 1984b: 9)

At this point, continues Pateman, we plunge right into the consideration of the role of ambiguity in art. If the contextualist position is right, then if we see St Theresa aright, there is no ambiguity in her facial expression: labelling the context as religious determines the expression as 'non-orgasmic ecstasy'. Against this, however, it could be argued that at the very least the secular perception of the facial expression is in some sense available in the religious context.

I would go further and argue that the secular perception of St Theresa's facial expression is undoubtedly available in the religious context. Lacan's view that it is an equivalent for secular orgasm is by no means pedestrian but surely the most likely and honest interpretation. Put differently, from what criterion other than the experiential do we interpret such an expression on the face of a young woman – surely not from the perspective of having personally witnessed a variety of female saints in religious ecstasy? (It might be noted, in passing, that certain contemporaries of Bernini criticized the sculpture as depicting a 'Venus'.)

It seems to me, then, that those who insist we should perceive St Theresa in a purely religious context, are subscribing to a thinly veiled form of propaganda. That is, a 'religious' interpretation does not so much guide our secular interpretation of the sculpture as manipulate it through half-truths. It is, therefore, not so much a case of our secular perception being available in the religious context as that the foundation of the religious context is inextricably bound to the secular one.[7]

Similarly, I would argue that our response to Maffei's *Judith* is not primarily governed by whether we know it to be a picture of Judith with the head of Holofernes or Salome with the head of John the Baptist. After all, we have no way of knowing what these remote biblical protagonists looked like – and neither did Maffei. Equally, we have no certain knowledge that they in fact existed or that a series of events were performed in their lives which culminated in a scene such as the one portrayed by Maffei.

In this light, Panofsky's insistence that our intuitively related response to *Judith* requires guidance, through recourse to iconological interpretation, becomes highly questionable.[8] That is, he is asking us to alter our intuitive understanding of a picture of a woman holding the decapitated head of a man by referring to a form of myth based in literary conjecture.[9] Yet surely few would argue that our correct response to literary interpretations of historical events requires qualification through recourse to visual means?

6.4 PRE-ICONOGRAPHICAL AND ICONOGRAPHICAL DESCRIPTIONS AS A SYMPTOM OF CEREBRAL SPECIALIZATION

Panofsky argues that pre-iconographical descriptions concern themselves with the 'natural' meanings and related expressive qualities found in works of visual art. This approach shares aspects in common with the way in which I have argued that the right hemisphere processes pictures; that is, it automatically and intuitively responds to our experientially derived but non-discursive understanding of a picture's referents. An iconographical approach to art, however, which implies a highly conceptualized and discursive understanding of art, possibly shares aspects in common with the way in which the left hemisphere processes phenomena. An important dimension to this view is substantiated by Gazzaniga and LeDoux's interpretation of the classic distinction between the recognition and recall of information (alluded to in the introduction and in chapters 2, 4, and 5).

Drawing from their lateralization research, Gazzaniga and Le-Doux argue that a dynamic view of how the brain manages the enormous task of storing various aspects of life in a readily accessible fashion involves the idea that experience is multi-dimensionally coded and recorded in memory. However, the memory

121

systems that store information do not necessarily communicate with each other and the verbal memory system may not be included at all. (This view shares aspects in common with Fodor's encapsulating *transducer* systems as reviewed in chapter 4.4.) Regarding the exclusion of the verbal system, we find:

> An example here comes from the common experience of being able to find one's way home from a new place even though the verbal system was engaged (say, through conversation) during the entire experience with the new route. If called upon to state the way, the verbal system could not do it. Yet, once on the way, the critical roads are recognized, and the proper choices for direction are made.
>
> (Gazzaniga and LeDoux 1978: 159)

The reason that this (modular) view of memory has been inadequately investigated, however, is because the memory mechanism that psychologists have been studying 'ad nauseam' is the verbal processing system.[10] And yet:

> What if this is but one of the systems of memory and, while it is working away, simultaneous activity is going on in several other nonverbal systems which have gestures or movements as their own modes of response ... If such an arrangement exists ... then one can indeed look at an embarrassingly huge number of previous studies on human memory and come to some unique conclusions about their meaning.
>
> (Gazzaniga and LeDoux 1978: 135–6)

It is argued that, adopting this view, the classic distinction between recognition and recall (that a person can recall only a small part of a body of information, whereas a great deal more can be recognized) immediately dissolves. According to the present model, the recall phase calls only upon the verbal system for response but it reports only a small amount of information because it has a limited capacity. When the recognition phase is introduced, however, all the information that the multiple nonverbal systems have stored can be reported, making the entire system more resourceful.

It seems to me that this version of the recognition phase could relate to Panofsky's view that pre-iconographical descriptions are concerned with the natural meanings and related expressive qualities found in visual art and also to my own that picture perception is an essentially non-discursive, right-hemisphere associated process involving intersensorial perception. Gazzaniga and LeDoux's version of the recognition phase can therefore be added to what has been so far concluded to produce schema 7.

Schema 7

recognition phase → pre-iconographical perception → intersensorially mediated memory experience of picture's phenomenal referents → right hemisphere amodal control mechanism → response

If the recognition phase relates to pre-iconographical perception and right-hemisphere processing, it could follow that iconography proper relates to left-hemisphere processing and the recall phase – given that recall calls upon the *verbal* system for response and that iconographical analysis presupposes a familiarity with specific themes or concepts transmitted through *literary* sources acquired by reading and oral tradition. In other words, I am suggesting that *recognition* can be equated with a pre-iconographical understanding and right-hemisphere function and *recall* with an iconographical understanding and left-hemisphere function. Therefore, when we *recognize* a picture this implies that it is understood in terms of our experientially derived and essentially non-discursive understanding of the world. When we *recall* a picture, we relate it to our conceptualized, linguistically formulated knowledge typically structured by others.[11]

Although verbally recalled knowledge may be capable of affecting our more intuitively derived (nonverbal) relations to art works, this does not mean that these respective 'ways of knowing' are mutually compatible or readily 'inter-translatable', and therefore 'knowable' – in fact, inherent in Panofsky's definition of iconography is the implication that they are not. Knowledge recalled thus exists to 'correct' an experientially derived understanding of art, a process developed by the art historian, who:

will do his best to familiarize himself with the social, religious and philosophical attitudes of other periods and countries, in order to correct his own subjective feeling for content ...
when he does all this, his aesthetic perception as such will change accordingly.

(Panofsky 1955: 17)

From a neuropsychological perspective, this view implies that the left hemisphere intervenes to insist on the pre-eminence of its particular way of knowing to the exclusion of all others. This hypothesis is substantiated by Gazzaniga and LeDoux's proposal that, although we possess multiple nonverbal memory systems, 'a case can be made that the entire process of maturing in our culture is the process of the verbal systems trying to note and eventually control the behavioural impulses of the many selves that dwell inside of us' (1978: 161).

This does not mean that the verbal system's attempt to control all other impulses necessarily results in a more certain knowledge of the world, however. As we saw in relation to P.S., his verbal system's tendency to rationalize resulted in it *confabulating* reasons for his right-hemisphere response to pictorial information. I return to the implications of this type of behaviour in the next chapter. For the present it is sufficient to note that we can now talk about the implication of two neuropsychologically defined ways of information processing competing to process a common stimuli form, the representational visual image.

6.5   TRANSLATABILITY AND THE VISUAL IMAGE

By drawing attention to the views of Panofsky in the light of those of Pateman, and attempting to contextualize them within a neuropsychological framework, I have raised the question of how *desirable* it is that our relations to certain works of visual art should be influenced by linguistically formulated knowledge. I shall conclude this chapter by examining a perhaps even more relevant (hermeneutic) issue, namely, how *possible* it is to linguistically account for these relations.

The most important question to ask is: how possible is it to successfully linguistically translate our pre-iconographic relations to visual art? The logical point here is that, unless it is possible to plausibly linguistically translate at this basic level, then the hermeneutic relevance of the ensuing levels within Panofsky's hierarchy surely become suspect. Panofsky himself might be seen as drawing attention to this point when he says, 'It is obvious that a correct iconographical analysis presupposes a correct identification of the motifs. If the knife which enables us to identify a St Bartholomew is not a knife but a corkscrew, the figure is not a

St Bartholomew' (1955: 30).

There might initially appear to be no problem here because, if pictures are perceived in virtue of their iconicity, no difficulty should be experienced in recognizing representations of knives or other miscellaneous forms found in pictures. There is, however, an important distinction between non-discursively identifying such forms and relating to their expressional qualities (pre-iconographic *perception*) and, beyond simply naming these forms, translating this process into language (pre-iconographic *description*). I can surely intuitively identify and relate to the expressional qualities suggested by the forms in Goya's *3rd May 1808* but would experience great difficulty in verbally describing the effects (and affects) of this perception (Figure 11). Regarding the difficulties involved in verbally describing such pre-iconographically associated responses, however, Panofsky is silent.

But here we can turn to Gombrich (1978) who confronts (although does not resolve) this central issue translation. Referring to some apples in a still life by Cézanne, Gombrich freely acknowledges that they 'say' infinitely more than can be summed up in words of any kind: 'This unique character of personal expression makes it quite untranslatable into words' (99). Gombrich continues by arguing that this 'notorious difficulty' (of translation) has less to do with art than with language, however, because neither a real apple nor one by Cézanne can ever be exhaustively described for the simple reason that varieties of apples are infinite but the number of words in any language is strictly finite. In so far as painting is something like a language, however, the limits of its translatability are of a different character and lie in the difficulty of finding clear and unambiguous terms for each of the possibilities the artist selected or rejected.[12] Because these terms cannot be at hand in everyday life, however, all the critic can do is to 'search for equivalent gamuts that allow him to convey his meaning through metaphor and analogy' (100).

In this way Gombrich unsuccessfully attempts to avoid his 'notorious difficulty' of translation by entering into areas even more epistemologically problematic. That is, having maintained that the (painted) representational image is untranslatable into words, he nonetheless assumes that certain aspects of artistic activity (the possibilities the artist rejected or selected) can be unambiguously explained through metaphor and analogy. The logical inference

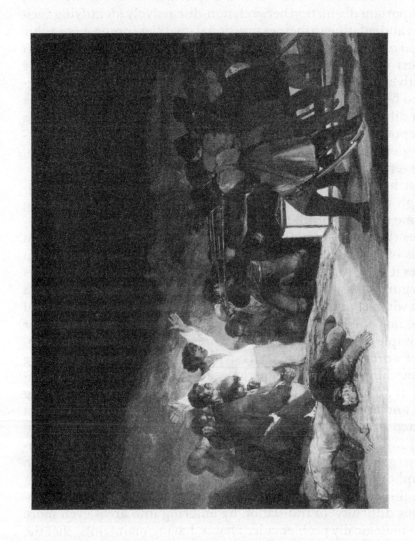

Figure 11 Francisco de Goya (1746–1828) *3rd May 1808*, canvas, 266 × 345 cm

Source: Prado, Madrid

is that art theoreticians must be capable of reading artists' minds through the vehicle of their work and thereafter be capable of communicating their findings through much debated forms of language study. In this way, we arrive at the following *non sequitur*: forms and their expressive qualities (a pre-iconographic perception of Cézanne's apples, for example) cannot be successfully linguistically translated because of the finiteness of words. Nonetheless, the intentions governing the artist's pictorial construction of forms and their expressive qualities can be successfully described through metaphor and analogy. That is, language so formulated can unambiguously account for why certain forms and their expressive qualities were selected in the first instance.

At this point we are surely entitled to ask: are Gombrich's equivalent (linguistic) gamuts truly equivalent or do they in fact constitute a semantically autonomous sign system capable of forming nothing more than a lengthy *anchorage* to direct or misdirect, as the case may be, our relations to the representational visual image?[13]

Here, we are not simply generalizing about the scope and limits of language (cf. Wittgenstein 1921) but talking about how possible and therefore plausible it is for one evolved symbol system to explicate an equally evolved but disparate one. That is, when referring to linguistic descriptions of certain classes of visual imagery, it has to be asked how hermeneutically valid is the proposition presented in schema 8.

Schema 8

real world phenomena → its (iconic) *re*presentation in the
form of selected marks (the artist's intention) arranged in
accordance with certain pictorial laws → the (iconic) representation's linguistic *re*presentation in the form of selected
words (the art theoretician's intention) arranged in accordance with syntactical laws → the role of the percipient as
reader of the syntax 'correcting' his role as *perceiver* of the
iconic representation.

Given that Gombrich acknowledges (but quickly attempts to bypass) the difficulties involved in linguistically translating even the simplest of represented forms (apples), the short answer to my original question is that his 'equivalent linguistic gamuts' surely do constitute a semantically autonomous sign system. The reason that (verbal) language cannot adequately account for the representational visual image has nothing to do with the finiteness of words, however. If this were the case then it would follow that were there sufficient words, no translation problem would exist. The fact of the matter is that Gombrich's 'notorious difficulty' is a qualitative and not a quantitative issue. His difficulty is centred around the communicative constraints inherent in the respective *forms* associated with language and image. Even with the best of intentions, therefore, when the art theoretician attempts to explicate the visual image, it is inevitably reconstructed in accordance with certain linguistic laws. In this way the visual image is not so much translated into language as *transformed* into a literary text.

From a neuropsychological perspective the implication is that the art theoretician's intention to explicate the representational visual image is typically symptomatic of the left (language) hemisphere's inherent tendency to attempt domination in processing information, regardless of its purpose or class. This tendency is reinforced by culture's more general but related ideological tendency to celebrate linguistic and rationalizing ways of knowing the world to the exclusion of all others.

As argued elsewhere, linguistic dominance is perhaps most easily accounted for by noting the inherent communicative natures and constraints associated with image- and language-making. That is, because language-making is inherently discursive it has the capacity to explicate the visual image, whereas because image-making is inherently non-discursive, it does not possess the same facility in regard to language. In other words, the hermeneutical flow is unidirectional.[14]

We are nonetheless still left with an anomaly of sorts. Although it may be that attempts to linguistically describe works of visual art inevitably confront translation difficulties, it is a practice which has a long history and continues to flourish unabated. In the next chapter I attempt to explain this persistence from a neuropsychologically substantiated viewpoint.

Chapter Seven

A TRANSFORMATIONAL THEORY OF AESTHETICS

7.1 INTRODUCTION

The stage has now been reached where the cognitive paradigms suggested by the neuropsychological data can be applied to form the basis for a new theory of aesthetic response. To the best of my knowledge no other aesthetic theories have been developed by drawing conclusions from neuropsychology, a comparatively recent development in the cognitive sciences, although phenomenological and psychological theories do, of course, have a substantial history.[1] This does not mean that my theory bears no relation to or has not benefited from other more traditional theories and, to emphasize this point, chapter 8 is dedicated to comparing my views with those of others.

Mine is not a general theory of aesthetic response in that it does not assume that a unifying thread exists connecting our various relations to distinct art forms, but is confined to the representational visual image and in particular to the 'art' image for reasons I explain in the next chapter. In this way I hope to have avoided the temptation of drawing conclusions for the arts in general on the basis of research relevant to perhaps only one or two of them (cf. Dickie 1974: 118–19).

Central to my theory is the view that our initial visual perceptions of the representational visual image result in it coming to be understood on a primarily non-discursive, right-hemisphere associated level of perception, as possessing a *full existential life* – that is, a life derived from our experiential understanding of an image's phenomenal referents.[2] This perception can result in the generation of a subtle state of emotional arousal that leads to an image appearing to possess what I term as *affective import*.

Although affective import is primarily right-hemisphere gener-

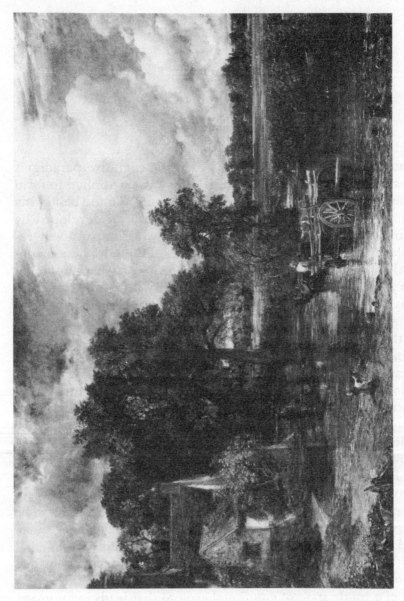

Figure 12 John Constable (1776–1837) *The Hay-Wain*, canvas, 130× 185 cm

Source: National Gallery, London

ated, it is communicated in holistic form to the left hemisphere, and in particular to its language centres, where it is discursively accommodated. This accommodation can result in affective import being associated with a certain kind of aesthetic experience and the image which appears to generate it being identified as the object of aesthetic experience.[3] Aesthetic experience is not viewed as something immutable, however, but as being subject to change in direct relation to the cognitive processes which constitute it.

Because the language centres possess no direct knowledge of the causes of this experience due to its association with right-hemisphere modes of cognitive processing, however, this has typically resulted in a consensus by aestheticians that it is an elusive and enigmatic phenomenon. Nonetheless, by and large, the enigma is not accepted but, on the contrary, prompts a variety of contemporary investigations into the nature of aesthetic experience and, when appropriate, its associated object, the representational visual image itself.

7.2   THE PARADOX OF PERCEPTUAL BELIEF HYPOTHESIS

In this section I introduce an hypothesis central to my theory. Because it proposes on several levels that our relations to the representational visual image involve profound psychological contradictions, I have termed it the *paradox of perceptual belief hypothesis*.

I have argued that we automatically process certain marks on a two-dimensional surface into appearing to constitute three-dimensional spatial relations and forms and this is a dominantly right-hemisphere associated activity (cf. chapters 2.4, 3.6, and 4.7). In this way, in virtue of their illusory three-dimensionality, certain marks psychologically suggest our visual-spatial understanding of phenomena. I have also argued that once these spatial relations and forms are perceived in virtue of their iconicity as having referents, our involved, experiential, but primarily non-discursive understanding of phenomena is activated (cf. chapters 4.7, 5.5, 6.4, and 6.5).

By way of illustration I suggest that, on perceiving Constable's *The Hay-Wain*, our attentions quite intuitively 'roam into' the illusory space and time continuum its visual planes, volumes, and distances, propose (Figure 12). As this process develops we quickly and effortlessly encounter known forms that become existentially significant because they release involved memory information pertaining to their referents. A cognitive 'journey' of *The Hay-Wain* might thus begin by our encountering its dog on the apparently solid ground of the nearby bank, its head turned toward the wain. Because we perceive that the greater part of the wain's wheels are visible (they are not submerged), we probably recognize that this part of the stream must be little more than ankle deep.[4] Our attentions may then be drawn 'beyond' the wain to the large expanse of field, its relative scale indicated by the diminutive trees in the distance compared to the size of those in the foreground; or they may be drawn 'upwards' to the large expanse of sky with its billowing clouds, their form and direction of movement implying the existence of a prevailing wind (cf. chapters 4.3, 5.2, and 5.5).

In this way, representational images can be understood as visual-spatial stimuli forms which automatically release complex, primarily non-discursive but specific memory information, thereby affording them a *full existential life*. It has to be emphasized, however, that this life is necessarily as illusory as the two-dimensional forms which constitute it. In virtue of their illusory three-dimensionality, therefore, certain visual marks *psychologically* suggest our involved visual-spatial and experiential relations to the phenomenal world, yet in virtue of their *phenomenal* two-dimensionality they necessarily remain distinctly apart from it. From this, I suggest that the instant we (involuntarily) mentally 'reconstitute', and therefore cognitively transform, certain marks on a two-dimensional surface into illusory spatial relations and forms, we experience a profound, but not readily linguistically introspectible, *paradox of perceptual belief*. (Both Gombrich and Wollheim recognize the possibility of this paradox, Wollheim having recently commented upon it at length in terms of 'twofoldness' cf. Wollheim 1987: 46–7 and 72–5.)

Thus, on one level of perception, we typically believe that the spatial relations and forms suggested by visual representations are mere illusions – we are not easily fooled, except in certain cases of *trompe-l'œil*, into believing that they possess in any phenomenal sense an existential life. On another level of perception, however, this belief is contradicted by the fact that their existential life continues to be experienced in what can be best described as an *equivocal reality*.[5] That is, a psychologized existential reality which, once activated, persists even when information from the same (rep-

132

resentational) source and inputted through the same (visual) modality which activated it, simultaneously contradicts its existence. *The Hay-Wain's* dog, stream, wain, field, sky, etc. do not relapse into abstraction because of our better (visually-derived) understanding that they are mere *illusions* – for example, that the perspective point suggested by the picture does not alter relative to our own movement as percipients rooted in the 'real world', and so forth (cf. chapter 6.3).

(And here it can be noted that the effects of equivocal reality are typically compounded if the representational image happens to be a *painting*. This is because, on the one hand, the artist's skill and control of the medium typically presents us with a heightened visual reality which is often, in one sense, more 'real' than visual reality itself, a point I return to in chapter 8. On the other hand, our better knowledge informs us that the illusion perpetrated has been artfully constructed from nothing except the artist's capacity to express his or her intentions through the medium of paint on an initially blank canvas.)

The reason for the (psychological) persistence of equivocal reality has already been substantiated from a neuropsychological perspective in this book and there is, therefore, no need to again discuss it at length. It is sufficient to note my argument that the same right-hemisphere associated paradigm which independently evolved to enable our species to instantly draw conclusions from our visual-spatial perceptions of the phenomenal world is automatically activated in its entirety by its iconic representation. In spite of our understanding that the visual-spatial and existential life of an image is mere illusion, therefore, this is insufficient to negate certain innately determined or biologically 'hardwired' responses which it activates as a special class of symbol form (cf. chapters 3.6 and 4.7, for example).

7.3 THE EXPECTATIONS AND RESPONSE TENDENCIES ACTIVATED BY VISUAL IMAGERY

I have argued that our capacity to recognize spatial relations and forms in the phenomenal world is not a passive process but evolved to enable us to *act* upon information (cf. chapters 3.6, 4.6, and 5.2). This process would have included what I term *primary expectations*, by which I mean expectations related to characteristics, visual-spatial or otherwise, we refer to on encountering an object or event to facilitate its identity. For example, included in our primary expectations of a suspended darkish mass, once conjectured to be a cloud, is the quality of movement. If the suspended mass confirms this expectation (it moves), this concomitantly confirms its holistic identity (this appears to be a cloud, we expect it to move, if it does it is a cloud). Expectations relevant to our visual perceptions of a certain animal form, once conjectured to be a dog, could include one of its auditory characteristics, *barking* (this appears to be a dog, in certain circumstances we expect it to bark, if it does it is a dog), and so forth (cf. chapter 1, notes 4 and 7, and chapter 4.2).

To have been of any practical use, primary expectations would have evolved in conjunction with certain response tendencies activated by conclusions drawn from these expectations. On confirmation in virtue of its kinetic properties that a certain darkish mass is in fact a cloud, a response tendency might be to shelter if it is believed to be a *rain* cloud. On an auditory percept confirming that a certain animal form is a dog, this could activate an evasive response tendency if the bark is aggressive, and so forth. (In this way, intersensorial perception and the expectations it gives rise to afford us a maximum grasp of a situation, etc. (cf. chapter 4.6).

From this it follows that related expectations and response tendencies apply, although typically in weakened form, to our perceptions of the world visually *re*presented. (This, taking into account my proposition in chapter 4.7 that the same right-hemisphere associated paradigm enabling us to draw conclusions from our visual-spatial perceptions of the phenomenal world is automatically activated in its entirety on our encountering its representation, and my related proposition in this chapter regarding the implications of a representation possessing a full existential life.) It might be, then, that our biologically determined and perhaps experientially reinforced understanding of Boucher's *Reclining Girl* produces sexual expectations, related response tendencies, and so forth (thereby substantiating Gombrich's view that the aim of 'erotic nudes' displayed on the covers and pages of magazines on sale in our cities is to produce the maximum permitted effect (cf. chapter 6.2).

In keeping with the origins of our understanding of a representation's existential life, however, this does not mean that a

majority of such expectations and response tendencies (because of
their right-hemisphere associations) are readily linguistically introspectible, although we may continue to feel their effects. We
have thus seen Gazzaniga and LeDoux hypothesize that non-verbal
mental modules can remember events, store affective reactions to
those events, and respond to stimuli associated with a particular
memory (cf. chapters 4.6, 5.6, and 6.4). Gazzaniga hypothesized
more recently:

> A response tendency, a decision for action on the part of a
> nonverbal mental module, is not unconscious. It is very con-
> scious, very capable of effecting action. One of its features,
> that it cannot internally communicate with the dominant
> hemisphere's language and cognitive system, should not find
> it being characterized as 'unconscious'.
>
> (Gazzaniga 1985: 117)

It is nonetheless clear that expectations and response tendencies
activated by an image's existential life cannot be resolved in terms
of the image itself. While the stream and billowing clouds in *The
Hay-Wain* may suggest expectations related to movement and *Reclining Girl* activate certain sexual response tendencies, these
necessarily remain psychological and potential. This suggests that
once the existential life of a visual representation activates certain
expectations and response tendencies which it cannot phenomenally resolve, this has the subsequent and paradoxical psychological
effect of its existential life being understood as *deficient*. Refer to
schema 9.

Schema 9

illusory spatial relations and forms recognized → activates
involved memory traces of an image's referents → image
perceived as possessing an existential life → activation of
expectations and response tendencies associated with this
existential life → realization that → image cannot resolve its
associated expectations and response tendencies → image
subsequently perceived as deficient.

It should be emphasized that I am not arguing that on perceiving
The Hay-Wain, for example, because of the 'real life' expectations
it activates, we expect it to 'magically' burst into activity: its stream

to flow and gurgle, clouds to drift across the sky and its horse-drawn cart to trundle. It is rather a case of the existential life associated with the representational visual image organizing our primarily right-hemisphere associated expectations and response tendencies on a non-discursive level of understanding and, because these cannot be resolved in terms of the image itself, this affects our subsequent perceptual and aesthetic relations, as we shall see presently.

7.4 THE INCOMPLETE IMAGE

I begin this section by reviewing the (mentalistic) hypothesis developed by Mandler (1975) regarding the consequences of interrupted plans and actions and subsequently show how it can help to explain the nature of our relations to the representational visual image.[6]

Mandler argues that if an expected system of events is in some way *interrupted* we subsequently attempt to *complete* the originally expected system, and in this way, 'All that is implied by the notion of interruption is that an organized response is "interrupted" whenever its completion is physically blocked or temporarily delayed – for whatever reason' (154). And regarding completion we find, 'Once an organized response has been interrupted, it is assumed that the tendency exists for completion for so long as the situation remains essentially unchanged' (154). And regarding the persistence of the need to complete:

> Completion can be derived from the continued functioning
> of some cognitive parallel of the overt organized response. If
> at the time of interruption, the sequential order of the or-
> ganized sequence has been laid down centrally, then the
> uncompleted part of the sequence will persist at the cognitive
> level as a plan (cf. Miller *et al.* 1960) even though the inter-
> ruption may disrupt the overt sequence.
>
> (Mandler 1975: 158)

Once the 'blocking agent' (which causes the interruption) has been removed, however, the original overt sequence can continue from the point of interruption and follow the isomorphic plan representing the original expected system.

Completion is not always possible along the lines of the original organized response, however, and when this occurs it results in a 'response substitution' which is described as, 'sequence completion by other organized sequences that are, more or less, specific to the interrupted sequence' (156). [A child is eating an ice-cream and some way through this process its organized response to consume all of it is interrupted because the ice-cream is dropped. The uncompleted part of this sequence persists at a cognitive level as a plan so that the child seeks its completion by attempting to buy another. But it is discovered that no more ice-cream is available so that the child has to make do with a 'response substitution' by buying another like product instead.]

One of the major consequences of interruption is that it leads to states of arousal followed by emotional behaviour, particularly if the original organized response cannot be completed in terms of other sequences specific to the original organized response:

> I suggest that the interruption of an organized response produces a state of arousal that, in the absence of completion or substitution, then develops into one or another emotional expression, depending on the occasion of the interruption.
> Thus interruption may lead to expressions of fear, anger, surprise, humor, or euphoria, depending entirely on factors *other than the interruption itself*.
>
> (Mandler 1975: 159)

[After dropping the ice-cream the child cannot obtain another or even a like product and this results in emotional behaviour such as a tantrum.]

Mandler continues by proposing that essentially the same arguments applying to the interruption of organized behaviour or action sequences apply to the interruption of mental structures:

> Given that a particular environmental input activates a specific organization, we assume that that structure determines the individual's perception and evaluation of the environment. A new input that activates a new structure may be interrupting if the new structure is incompatible with the old, or if it contradicts the operation of the old structure or, more generally, if it provides inputs that are not manageable (i.e. cannot be assimilated by the existing structure).
>
> (Mandler 1975: 169–70)

Mandler's contention that a new (cognitive) structure activated by a new input may be interrupting because it contradicts the operations of old structures, is relevant to the underlying cognitions implied by my paradox of perceptual belief hypothesis. With particular reference to schema 9, therefore, I suggest that Mandler's 'old structure' can be readily substituted by my 'image perceived as possessing an existential life'. This perception is subsequently interrupted by the 'new structure' one – 'image cannot resolve its associated expectations and response tendencies'.

Therefore, because of the complex memory information released by our initially visual perceptions of an image, it is consequently understood as possessing a full existential life, thus organizing our expectations, response tendencies, and so forth. Our initially visual perceptions of *Reclining Girl*, for example, may organize expectations and response tendencies in such a way that we become sexually aroused, feel desire, and so forth. This response tendency is subsequently interrupted, however, by our 'new structure' understanding that this response cannot 'complete' in terms of its activating stimuli, the image itself, because of its two-dimensional illusory nature.

Although it may be that our expectations and organized responses, initially activated by our visual perceptions of an image, are interrupted by our subsequent understanding of its existential deficiency, this does not mean that the image relapses into abstraction thereby dissolving the interruption process. (That is, if it relapsed into abstraction it would no longer psychologically possess an existential life and therefore no longer instigate existentially related expectations, response tendencies, and so forth.) This is because we are referring to an innately determined psychologized existential reality which, once activated, persists regardless of incoming visual information simultaneously contradicting its existence. In principle, from this it follows that an image could continue to activate expectations, organized responses and interruptions for the duration of its perception.

Given for the moment that this is the case, then in terms of Mandler's hypothesis it follows that, concomitant with the interruption process, a tendency for completion exists for the duration that the existential life of an image continues to be perceived (taking into account that a tendency for completion exists for as long as the situation remains essentially unchanged and that a picture is materially unchangeable). The difficulty here, however, is that the very cause of the interruptions ensures the impossibility of their completion, namely, once again, the representational image's material immutability.

From this it follows that a representation's inability to complete (the 'blocking agent' is not removed) the expectations, response tendencies and interruptions it so readily activates, generates a search for a 'response substitution'. But the difficulty here is that under normal circumstances there are no overt ways of substituting for the expectations and response tendencies our existential understanding of an image activates. (But see chapter 5.4, regarding how children's relations to the representational visual image can include overt responses to the associations and expectations it activates.)

It would appear, then, we are at that stage where, if Mandler's hypothesis is true, in the absence of completion or substitution, an organized response can lead to an emotional expression of some sort.

7.5   CATHECTIC TRANSFERENCE

I argue in this section that our existentially derived relations to the representational visual image can result in emotional responses which, because they cannot be overtly expressed, produce emotional tensions. These tensions are subsequently released, in virtue of *cathectic transference*, to transform our perceptions of the representational image.

Given Mandler's hypothesis and that there typically exist no overt ways of substituting for the expectations and possible response tendencies our existential understanding of an image activates, then it follows that we become emotionally aroused. It also follows that this state is capable of producing emotional tensions which continue until such time as they are released and resolved through some form of emotional expression. The continuing difficulty, however, is that, as with response substitutions, there typically exist no readily available means of emotionally releasing the tensions our perceptions of an image might arouse. Several interrelated reasons for this are worth mentioning.

First, the nature of our expectations and response tendencies, because of their derivation in our right-hemisphere perceptions of an image, are not readily linguistically introspectible. This has the implication that the less discursively aware we are of the causes of the emotions within us the less able we are equipped to deal with them.

Second, the initial degree of emotional intensity produced by our (interrupted) responses to an *image* of the world, will in most instances be less strong than the one produced by the interruption of real life events. (This is consistent with my contention that the expectations and response tendencies associated with life situations apply in only *weakened* form to our relations to the representational visual image.) The point here is that in most circumstances the emotions activated by an image are insufficiently intense to trigger in a reflex fashion some form of emotional outburst, thereby dissolving them.

Third, even if this were the case, any such outburst would typically be inhibited by social pressures to conform. (It is worth noting, however, that Metz remarks that film spectators in small towns in France and Italy often find emotional release from their understanding of a film by rising from their seats, gesticulating and shouting to the hero, or insulting the 'bad guy' (1982: 101).)[7] In general, however, I suggest that our emotional responses to an image remain suppressed until they are afforded some form of less overt releasing agency.

Granted, then, that there typically exist no overt ways of releasing the emotions activated by our relations to an image, and given that it is incapable of material change, it could appear that we are faced with a tension ridden and circular 'cognitive impasse'. That is, taking into account my paradox of perceptual belief hypothesis, the emotions and tensions generated by our relations to an image, continue *ad infinitum*, or at least for the duration of its perception.

I suggest that the interruption process does, in fact, continue in a circular fashion for a short time (measured in perhaps seconds or less. See note 6 of my introduction to this book). Eventually, however, it is the image itself which (paradoxically) provides the substitutive vehicle capable of offering a form of emotional release, a way of (vicariously) completing the expectations, response tendencies and subsequent emotions and tensions it activates in virtue of its existential life. My reasoning here is that, with all possible overt forms of emotional release 'blocked', the release has to be effected by some form of paradigm shift, some form of *adaptive psy-*

chological change in the percipient. This is brought about by a concentrated psychological projection or *cathectic transference* of the emotions and tensions 'into' the one relevant outlet readily available to perception, *the representational visual image itself.* This transference has the subsequent effect of transforming the image into appearing to become 'psychologically energized', into appearing to possess what I term as *affective import.* This process is schematized in 10.

Schema 10

representational image with existential life → expectations
and response tendencies → cannot complete → image
perceived as existentially deficient → interruptions →
response substitutions which are subsequently 'blocked' →
emotional arousal/tensions → cannot be overtly released →
cathectic transference → image becomes substitutive vehicle
and is thereby perceived as possessing affective import

7.6 THE NATURE OF AFFECTIVE IMPORT

I have proposed that our initially visual perceptions of the representational visual image can trigger a complex series of cognitive transformations leading to it appearing to possess affective import. I have also proposed that affective import can come to be associated with aesthetic experience. I attempt to establish the possible nature of the relations between affective import and aesthetic experience in the next section and in chapter 8. I shall, however, first provide a working definition of affective import (because only then will it be possible to later compare it to more traditional views on the nature of aesthetic experience).

The first thing to establish is that, although a series of cognitive transformations can lead to the particular mental state I have described as affective import, this does not mean it is a stable, immutable, and a singular state which, once obtained, is incapable of change. In other words, I view affective import as being a *relative* mental state which plays nothing more nor less than a central part in a dynamic cognitive continuum. Therefore, although it may be that at an important stage in our perceptions of the representational image it appears to become 'psychologically energized', thereby possessing affective import, this does not mean that this state is necessarily sustained *ad infinitum* or that it is devoid of some of the former mental states and stages that helped to constitute it in the first instance.

I have argued that affective import fulfils an essentially compensatory function realized by a transference of emotion 'into' its object and cause – the representational image itself. Affective import does not therefore exist in isolation as a disembodied mental state but can be understood only in terms of its object, the one immutable, phenomenally constant component in the transformational process I have described. Although capable of generating complex mental changes in the percipient, the representational image does not itself change but remains materially constant thereby providing the perfect substitutive vehicle, the perfect catalyst for the release and 'funnelling' of emotion.

The way in which an image funnels emotion is in virtue of those very properties that, once having obtained an existential life, cause the emotion in the first instance – its visual properties. It is these that become 'psychologically energized' and imbued with an extraordinary or heightened *visual* significance.

I have emphasized 'visual' because at this advanced *adaptive* stage in the transformational process it would be psychologically inconsistent for a picture to continue to be perceived as possessing a *full* existential life – if it did then this would negate the essentially *compensatory* role of affective import. At this stage in the transformational process, then, a representation's full existential life is necessarily 'blocked' or *suppressed* from consciousness, leaving its visual properties as the primary focus of attention. This typically results in a tendency towards a detached exploration of these properties, that, once possessed of a full existential life, now necessarily appear strangely distanced or apart from it. In this way the quality of affective import might be compared to dream perception in which the dreamer, while perhaps vaguely aware that an unreality is being perpetrated, nonetheless remains entranced by it as if straddled between two perceptual realms subject to different laws (cf. Sartre 1948).

Although at this stage in the transformational process an image's full existential life may be 'blocked' from the percipient, the image does, then, retain the capacity to remind us of aspects of this life, in particular the visual nature of the phenomenal world. For example, that certain visual properties suggest a tree, clouds and a stream; others a horse and cart, and that these images collectively perceived suggest a country scene in the manner of *The Hay-Wain*. But it is now a scene that exists apart from phenomenal connotations in a psychological 'limbo' reminiscent of, but strangely divorced from, reality. It is as if the normally intersensorially perceived phenomenal world in all its complexity and implications has become concentrated into a 'visually encapsulated island', that is, one in which only things visual assume significance.

I am suggesting, then, that for compensatory and adaptive reasons, affective import is typically associated with a psychological 'distancing' from phenomenal events as pictorially alluded to, with the effect that the primarily visual nature of an image comes to appear extraordinarily significant.[8] Thus what begins as an existentially derived involvement in the representational visual image in virtue of its full existential life, (paradoxically) culminates in a necessary psychological suppression of this involvement with consequent cognitive and perceptual effects.

As I have implied, however, this does not mean that the percipient at all times remains psychologically distanced from the representation; put differently, the state of affective import is not necessarily sustained *ad infinitum* because of the suppressive processes I have described. It is sometimes the case that a representation's full existential life temporarily reasserts itself thereby (again) resulting in an (existentially derived) involvement with an image. Although this reassertion of involvement is necessarily soon suppressed in order to maintain a cognitive equilibrium (i.e. in order to fulfil its compensatory role as a substitutive vehicle), at times the percipient may rapidly alternate between the two mental states I have described, that is, essentially a practical and a trans-practical interest in the representational visual image (cf. Coleman 1983: 55).

7.7 AFFECTIVE IMPORT AS AESTHETIC EXPERIENCE

In this section I argue that, although affective import is primarily right-hemisphere generated, it is nonetheless communicated to the left-hemisphere associated language centres by means of an 'emotional aura'. This essentially left-hemisphere removed perception can result in a consensus that a certain mental state exists typically characterized as aesthetic experience.

In chapter 2.5 we saw Sperry *et al.* (1979) hypothesize that, in the case of the subject L.B., the left hemisphere became aware of unilaterally right-hemisphere registered and processed pictorial information by means of an 'emotional aura' that spread through the brain stem systems. With appropriate prompting from the examiner this enabled the subject to 'guess' the nature of the information, as evidenced by its (eventual) linguistic identification. From this result it was argued that common experience suggests that such auras play an important orientational role in normal brain function; mnemonic retrieval, for example. I also referred in this section to tests conducted by Gazzaniga and LeDoux (1978) when it appeared that unilaterally right-hemisphere registered and processed pictorial information of an emotional and conative class 'leaked', in a directionally specific manner, to the left hemisphere.

Given my contention that an image's affective import is dominantly right-hemisphere generated, it is reasonable to hypothesize that it is communicated to the language centres in something like the way described above. That is, it spreads from the right hemisphere, via the corpus callosum and lesser brain communication pathways, after which it is registered in holistic form by the language centres.

(It should be emphasized that I am not suggesting it is a case of pictorial information being exclusively registered by the right hemisphere and it subsequently spreading to the left in some form. Clearly, such is the nature of our visual system that pictorial information is processed by both hemispheres cf. chapter 1.2. What I have argued is that the right hemisphere processes information *differently* to the left. Therefore, because of its close evolutionary links with directly and intuitively interpreting the phenomenal world, it relates strongly to an image's existential life. It is the consequences of these relations, for the reasons described, that spread in holistic form to the language centres, cf. chapter 3.6 and most of chapter 4, for example. In this way the language centres experience in removed and abstract form the consequences of right-hemisphere associated perceptions and cognitions of the representational image.)

I also suggest that, in advance of merely passively registering affective import, the language centres typically recognize it as a special (an extraordinary) kind of experience which is subsequently often characterized as 'aesthetic'. My reasoning here is that if our right-hemisphere perceptions of the representational image activate complex cognitions of the order described, then this is an habitual process whose effects recurrently spread to and are consequently recognized by the language centres. Refer to schema 11.

Schema 11

representational visual image → RH cognitions → affective import, i.e. image becomes psychologically energized → emotional aura communicated via the corpus callosum, etc. → registered by left-hemisphere language centres → LH cognitions → affective import characterized as aesthetic experience.

Although it may be that affective import is registered and characterized by the language centres as a kind of aesthetic experience, this does not mean they have any direct knowledge of its causes. On the contrary, given my arguments regarding the right-hemisphere generated and essentially non-discursive nature and origins of affective import, the indications are this is unlikely to be the case. This view is substantiated by the fact that, although there may be a consensus that aesthetic experience is of a special kind, it tends to be widely acknowledged that it is an elusive and enigmatic phenomenon. We thus find Diffey proposing:

> There is a well-established literature in philosophy on aesthetic experience and *prima facie* it seems that aesthetic experience is a topic about which we can theorize and make significant statements. Yet what are we talking about when we talk about aesthetic experience? It is a shocking admission to have to make, but I have to confess that I do not know. At the very least I find that the notion of aesthetic experience is unclear. I, or perhaps we, since I do not believe that I am alone in this matter, have no clear grasp of the notion.
>
> (Diffey 1986: 3)

Alternatively, we find Hosper's essentially defensive declaration:

> The starting point of all philosophy of art is the fact of esthetic experience.... And the first point it is necessary to make about esthetic experience is that there is such a thing: that is to say, that there is a kind of experience which,

though not completely isolated from the rest of our experience, is sufficiently distinct from it to deserve a special name, 'esthetic'.

(Hospers 1976: 3)

However, this is soon followed by: 'I have not defined the esthetic attitude. I do not think it possible to define it in other words. Like all expressions which refer to experience or states of feeling, one must have had the experience to know what it is like' (7).

Hospers therefore begins by insisting upon the existence of aesthetic experience as a distinct 'way of knowing' but hastily follows this with a disclaimer of sorts: it is something that can only be experienced. If we have not had this experience then we simply do not know what it is like and there is, therefore, no point in attempting to define it in 'other words'. (This view clearly echoes Gombrich's regarding our response to a still life by Cézanne. We thus saw Gombrich propose that it 'says' infinitely more than can be summed up in words of any kind; that 'This unique character of personal expression makes it quite untranslatable into words'. Cf. chapter 6.6).

We find Lindauer pointing out in a more general vein:

The topic of aesthetics, central though it may be to the psychology of art, cannot be easily defined. Its diverse meanings and uses led Nunally (1977) to declare that 'one must stand in awe of a term that covers so much'.... Not even its spelling (aesthetics or esthetics) is certain.

(Lindauer 1981: 29)

It is consequently not surprising that it should be said, as Dickie does, that, 'the expression "aesthetic experience" is used with great frequency by aestheticians, sometimes without any clear meaning attached to it and almost always without a precise idea as to the nature of the referent of the expression' (1974: 182).

Diffey, Hospers, Lindauer, Nunally, and Dickie are by no means isolated in their view that aesthetic experience is an enigmatic phenomenon. I suggest, therefore, that whereas a majority of aestheticians are ready to acknowledge the existence of aesthetic experience and that it is often prompted by works of art, not unlike the subject L.B.'s response to unilaterally right-hemisphere registered and processed information, great difficulty is experienced in verbally characterizing it.

It thus has to be assumed that aesthetic experience is a real phenomenon felt by aestheticians and non-aestheticians alike. Because aesthetics is a discursive discipline, however, the onus is clearly on its practitioners to comment upon aesthetic experience (given that the nature of the aesthetic is the core of aesthetics). But then I have argued that a certain type of experience sometimes defined as 'aesthetic' is essentially non-discursive because it reaches the language centres in holistic form after transfer from the right hemisphere. If I am right in this hypothesis then it follows that when attempts are made to linguistically introspect the nature of the experience the aesthetician is faced with a neuropsychologically based epistemological dilemma. That is, faced with the difficulties involved in explicating an essentially biologically removed perception in the sense that the left-hemisphere associated language centres have to attempt to explain, in their own terms, an essentially right-hemisphere processed and generated phenomenon.

(If I am correct in these assumptions, then one way in which we can think of the brain's operations is in terms of its localized parts functioning as either a *sender* or *receiver* of information. Incoming information, relayed to the brain via the senses, is initially processed by those parts most suited to a particular task. The information may then be sent to other biologically distinct parts of the brain capable of receiving it, but probably only in holistic form. Whenever possible, the newly received information is subsequently *re-processed* in accordance with the capacities associated with these parts, and so forth. In this way, incoming information is successively filtered and transformed in virtue of its journey through distinct mental systems.)

7.8 'TALKING ABOUT' THE REPRESENTATIONAL VISUAL IMAGE

I have argued that a certain kind of experience, sometimes described as aesthetic, is of an essentially non-discursive origin. If I am right in this view, then when this kind of experience is associated with works of art it follows that, like the aesthetician, the art theoretician is faced with a discursive dilemma centred around inferring from insufficient units of information. The theoretician thus possesses a unit which informs of the (holistic) existence of aesthetic experience and a unit which informs that this in some (causal) way relates to the object of aesthetic experience, for my purposes the representational visual image. What is not possessed, however, are those vital units of information which relate to the complex causes of aesthetic experience. Refer to schema 11. The theoretician is therefore in a situation which, in certain essential respects, parallels the one experienced by the commissurotomy subject P.S., examined by Gazzaniga and LeDoux (cf. chapters 2.5, 4.4, and 6.5).

It will be recalled that P.S. was asked to solve a problem on the basis of pictorial information unilaterally registered by both hemispheres. His left hemisphere thus possessed three units of information but lacked a vital fourth possessed by his right hemisphere which would have enabled his discursive (left-hemisphere) self to arrive at a correct solution. This situation did not, however, appear to present P.S. with any lasting difficulty because he (his discursive self) simply obviated the effects of those units of information to which he did not have discursive access and subsequently concentrated on interpreting those units to which he did. Although this cognitive strategy resulted in pure confabulation, its effects nonetheless appeared to perfectly satisfy the discursive needs of P.S.

I have returned to this clinical data because the strategy adopted by P.S. is often, in my view, symptomatic of the one adopted by the art theoretician on continually being prompted to accommodate the enigma of aesthetic experience within a discursive framework. That is, the theoretician eventually concentrates on those units of information relevant to aesthetic experience which are discursively accessible and which can therefore be discursively embellished upon. In this regard, the only readily available unit is the one whose paradoxical nature induces aesthetic experience in the first instance, the representational visual image itself.

In greater detail, the art theoretician's right-hemisphere associated perceptions of the representational image induce that particular mental state I have termed as affective import. This state is communicated in holistic form to the language centres where it is sometimes characterized as aesthetic experience. Such is the nature of this experience (it is enigmatic, it is different to ordinary experience, etc.) that it prompts comment in keeping with the language centre's biologically evolved tendency to rationalize and qualify information. But a real difficulty is experienced in this regard for the reasons I have described. At this advanced stage in the transformational process, therefore, I suggest that the theoretician is confronted with a 'cognitive impasse' (commenting upon the essentially non-discursive) subsequent to the one whose effects result in a certain kind of aesthetic experience in the first instance.

The way in which the theoretician often attempts to resolve this (new) impasse is by putting into effect a *secondary level of cathectic transference*. Thus, with direct access to vital units of information relevant to aesthetic experience 'blocked' from (discursive) consciousness, but still motivated by their effect, the theoretician, like P.S., has to re-channel energies. This re-channelling is effected by concentrating on seeing how the materially constant representational image, as the object of aesthetic experience, and the one unit of information readily available to perception, can be discursively accommodated. Put differently, the theoretician, like P.S., searches by way of a substitutive behaviour for ways of seeing how the representational visual image can be what I shall simply term *talked about*. In this regard, no great difficulty is experienced because of the surfeit of linguistically structured hermeneutic strategies developed over time to comment on the representational visual image (cf. chapter 6.4).

Talking about the representational image does not, of course, exist in isolation but, it has to be assumed, is produced to be assimilated by others thereby affecting their perceptions. Taking into account the theory of hemispheric specialization, this can be approached differently by saying that reference to at least certain linguistic descriptions of the visual image has the effect of producing a paradigm shift. That is, a shift *away* from percipients' right-hemisphere (direct, intuitive, recognitory) and towards their left-hemisphere (indirect, discursive, recall) associated ways of knowing the representational visual image. In this way, reference to *talking about* implies that a percipient is prone to think *about* the image in question by gathering all available linguistically imparted data relevant to its status, thereby inhibiting a more intuitive response.[9] Refer to schema 12.

I have argued in this section that the enigmatic nature of a certain kind of experience, sometimes described as aesthetic, can motivate the art theoretician to put into effect a *secondary level of cathectic transference*. This essentially adaptive and compensatory behaviour can result in *talking about*, often at length, the object of aesthetic experience, the representational visual image.

Schema 12

Art theoretician → RH way of knowing the representational image induces affective import which is → sometimes characterized by the LH as aesthetic experience → because the LH cannot (linguistically) introspect the nature of aesthetic experience but remains motivated by its effects, this results in → LH concentration on the object of aesthetic experience (the image itself) which results in it being *talked about* → reference to *talking about* results in a paradigm shift away from a RH (direct, intuitive, recognitory) and towards a LH (indirect, discursive, recall) way of knowing the representational visual image.

Sufficient has been said in this book regarding the desirability of referring to at least certain forms of discourse surrounding 'art' to avoid reiteration here (cf. chapter 6). It therefore only remains to say that, because *talking about* is viewed as being the conclusion of a chain of neuropsychologically associated mental processes initially caused by our right-hemisphere associated perceptions of the representational visual image, it exists as an integral part of my transformational theory and in part solves the problem suggested by the *causation issue* presented in section 2 of my introduction to this book.

7.9   THE MUNDANE REPRESENTED

I have argued that our relations to the representational image's existential (as distinct from exclusively visual) life can lead to an emotional response that results in affective import. This emphasis on the effects of an image's existential component could result in a misinterpretation of my theory, however. It could be thought that I have insufficiently distinguished between our responses to images of the world and the world itself. This could in turn lead to the conclusion that only those images whose referents are associated with strong emotional connotations (violent or sexual imagery, for example) are capable of triggering the processes I have described, resulting in affective import. The emphasis in this section is therefore on clarifying why it is that a wide variety of images are capable of generating this special kind of experience.

Of central importance to an understanding of my theory is

proper consideration of my argument that it is *not* our direct existentially derived relations to an image's referents that primarily cause an emotional response. This response is generated by what can be thought of as *second order* cognitive processes.

I have argued that, because of their catalytic nature, images can activate an existentially derived understanding of their referents and in this way they come to possess a full existential life. This understanding can in turn cause (in typically weakened form) certain relevant expectations and response tendencies (in spite of our better knowledge that images are mere illusions, etc.). It does not follow, however, that at this stage in our relations to the visual image we necessarily experience any obvious emotion. It is our subsequent *inability to respond* to (and therefore resolve) the expectations and response tendencies activated by an image that can result in a state of emotional arousal (cf. section 7.4). This state, with its accompanying tensions, is eventually suppressed, however, in virtue of cathectic transference, to affect our relations to the image (cf. sections 7.5 and 7.6).

Importantly, then, the psychological processes and effects that may result in an emotional response derived from our understanding of an image's full existential life, should not be confused with the response that may result on our encountering its referents in the phenomenal world. Our emotional response to an image is contingent upon tensions related to its (removed) capacity to visually suggest, but our *inability to respond*, to its full existential life – and not upon a *direct* emotional response to the subject represented.

It might be argued, however, that whereas images with overtly sensational connotations may be obviously capable of generating certain expectations and response tendencies because of our existentially derived understanding of their referents, this cannot be said to be true of a majority of images, that is, images of the mundane not normally associated with emotionally sensational connotations. If it cannot, then the implication is that only a minority of images are likely to cause significant emotional responses culminating in affective import.

However, given that from early childhood our developmental and intersensorially mediated experience of the world instils in us certain expectations and response tendencies, because these are typically caused by our relations to the mundane, does not indicate their psychological insignificance – on the contrary, their relations to the mundane indicates an habituation which *reinforces their place in our psychology*.

I have emphasized this point because, if an image refers us to mundane events in the world, these carry with them quite *definite* sequences of expectations and response tendencies. Consequently, if these are interrupted through our inability to respond, it follows that a *significant* level of emotional arousal ensues leading to affective import, etc.

In 'real life' circumstances this is unlikely to be the case simply because expectations and response tendencies, elicited by our relations to the mundane, are typically not interrupted but resolved. On encountering a phenomenal equivalent of *The Hay-Wain*, for example, this country scene's billowing clouds, stream, dog, and so forth, may all elicit certain expectations and response tendencies related to our understanding of movement. In addition, our (initially) visual perceptions of the scene as a whole may elicit a host of auditory expectations. Such expectations are typically resolved, however, because of the scene's existence in the continually unfolding phenomenal world. In this way the world, as distinct from the world *re*presented, typically provides insufficient grounds for the generation of affect import.

Chapter Eight

ART AND AESTHETIC EXPERIENCE

8.1 INTRODUCTION

Although there may be a consensus that aesthetic experience is an elusive phenomenon, as was suggested in the previous chapter, this does not mean that attempts have not been made to understand it or necessary conditions proposed for its existence. These conditions are by no means uniform, however, but often appear diametrically opposed so that, viewed collectively, it is not unusual for profound contradictions to exist between certain aesthetic theories.

For example, traditional but still influential philosophically and psychologically based theories which argue that aesthetic experience is generated by the percipient being in some way disinterested or 'psychically distanced' from the work of art (Bullough 1912; Osborne 1970; Hospers 1974; Stolnitz 1960, 1986) are challenged by phenomenological theories of the order proposed by Dewey (1934), Merleau-Ponty (1962, 1964), Dufrenne (1973), and Berleant (1970, 1986). Berleant, for example, argues that our aesthetic relations to works of art are generated not by being 'distanced' from them but in virtue of our very involvement.

And then there is the question of whether aesthetic experience is necessarily exclusively related to works of art or whether it is a type of experience that can be generated by a diversity of phenomena. Even if we confine the concept of aesthetic experience to our relations to works of art, however, this in turn raises the traditional and enormous problem, namely, What is art?

If we relate aesthetic experience to art, it is a question that needs to be taken seriously simply because, before aesthetic experience can be defined in terms of our experience of art, we need to be reasonably certain of what constitutes art in the first instance. The question is notoriously difficult to answer, however, not least because, as Hospers points out:

> The felt qualities of the experiences of various persons, even
> those thoroughly steeped in the arts, are extremely various.
> This is all the more so when we consider not only the variety
> of persons doing the experiencing, their diverse backgrounds
> and temperaments, but also the great differences in the
> artistic media, and the various genres of art within each
> medium, not to mention the even greater differences
> between our responses to art and our responses to nature.
>   (Hospers 1982: 360)

But even if we confine ourselves to understanding our relations
to art as associated with the representational visual image, as I have
done, this by no means solves the problem of What is art? The representational image is communicated to us through a variety of
visual media which daily proliferate in keeping with contemporary
technological means of production. How, then, are we to artistically
distinguish between the effects of different visual media, painting
as distinct from photography, for example? How are we to distinguish between Boucher's *Reclining Girl* and an image from *Playboy*,
or, for that matter, a contemporary piece of photographic 'eroti-
cism' by Robert Mapplethorpe?

Dickie, in his version of the institutional theory, might argue
that we cannot distinguish with certainty because even a medium
as traditional as painting comes to be a work of *art* only in so far
as certain people occupying certain socially identifiable positions
(the representatives of the art world) confer this status upon it (with
the implication that works of art are not necessarily possessed of
immutable universal qualities transcendent of time and place but
are, rather, subject to the dictates of the fashion of the time, cf.
Dickie 1974; Danto 1984; and for a criticism of Dickie's views, see
Wollheim 1987: 13–16).

And then Diffey has recently proposed that, although it may be
that aesthetic experience is traditionally associated with our relations to works of art, this is not necessarily desirable, because:

> We are always in danger of having this kind of identification
> exert a tacit influence over our thinking unless we are willing
> to face and confront the question explicitly and openly: what
> does aesthetic experience have to do with the experience of
> art. I therefore have a good deal of sympathy with Dickie's

proposal, *if* our interest is really in works of *art*, to drop talk about aesthetic experience, and to talk instead about our experience of works of art. We can then examine in an open way what it is to experience works of art without being confused or prejudiced by the body of work in philosophy which is devoted to the subject of aesthetic experience.

(Diffey 1986: 4)

Scruton, on the other hand, argues that if we wish to gain insights into the nature of aesthetic experience we should *not* concentrate on works of art, because, 'It has seemed to me more profitable to analyse the aesthetic experience itself, and in particular that central core of "imaginative attention" which interested Wittgenstein and Sartre' (1983: 13).

In relation to Diffey's views, however, the nature of aesthetic experience notwithstanding, we still remain with the question of by what criteria do we distinguish art from other other phenomena – and in relation to Scruton's views, the nature of art notwithstanding, with the question of by what criteria do we distinguish aesthetic experience from other (non-aesthetic) experience.[1]

Although there are clearly no easy answers to these questions, the emphasis in this chapter is on attempting to show that what can appear as marked differences between certain aspects of major aesthetic theories are (a) often partially explicable by viewing them as an emphasis on the different cognitive stages of the transformational processes I have described, and (b) result as a failure to take into account the different communicative constraints inherent in distinct art forms.

However, because aesthetic experience is tacitly associated with our relations to works of art, and because what constitutes art continues to be an issue central to aesthetics and the philosophy of art, I shall begin by saying something about its possible nature, whenever feasible confining my attentions to the representational visual image.

Finally, my references to certain aestheticians are not meant to be comprehensive in terms of either their views or the history of their discipline. I have, rather, selected from only aspects of those views which appear relevant to the thesis I have developed throughout this book.

8.2   ART AND THE REPRESENTATIONAL VISUAL IMAGE

Many years ago, as a graduate student of the Slade School in London, I produced a series of (art) works and attempted to sell them door-to-door in the wealthier boroughs. I was sometimes successful and in the course of my enterprise was often invited into the homes of potential buyers. On occasions this involved being shown works already acquired and usually prominently displayed. I mention this because many of these would probably have been considered 'banal' by those in some way professionally engaged in the art world and dismissed in no uncertain terms. And yet the owners were often effusive as to the quality of their acquisitions and exhibited responses traditionally associated with aesthetic experience.

Were, then, these collectors undergoing a genuine aesthetic experience in relation to their 'art' or were they simply misguided in their belief? Although this may appear to be an arrogant question to pose, it is nonetheless a relevant one if we subscribe to the view that aesthetic experience is exclusively generated by our relations to works of *art*. On this basis, many of my potential buyers, whatever *they* may have thought, were not having an *aesthetic* experience but some other kind. But by what criteria are we to differentiate our relations to art and other phenomena?

In relation to the representational visual image, perhaps the most logical way would be to begin by examining the implications of its visual characteristics: how convincingly Rembrandt can render the craggy flesh of old age, Poussin a sense of depth in his landscapes, or Holbein the minutiae of an object, for example. This is not, however, an approach typically favoured by aestheticians if we are to believe the recent views of Mitias:

> Of one thing, though, I am certain, *viz.*, it is extremely difficult, almost impossible, to define, or attempt to define, 'art' on the basis of observable or exhibited, property, or set of properties. And the aestheticians who constructed theories of art like Kant, Hegel, Schopenhauer, Croce, Collingwood, Santayana, Dewey, Fry, to mention just a few names, did not, I am certain, distinguish art works as a class on the basis of empirically observable properties, but on the basis of unexhibited properties, properties that come to life, fruition, or actualization in the aesthetic experience.
>
> (Mitias 1986: 52)

Not surprisingly, however, Mitias goes on to point out that this requires a clarification of what is meant by 'aesthetic' and then to hypothesize how Hospers might criticize his views:

But Hospers would object: if aesthetic qualities are essentially unexhibited, or, as you say, exist as a complex of potentialities in the art work, if they come to life and acquire existence and identity in an aesthetic experience, then we have no way to know either what makes art works *art* or aesthetic experience *aesthetic*, for the aesthetic experiences of the people who perceive and appreciate art works are, as we say, *diverse*; it is in principle extremely difficult for two or more individual percipients to have the same experience of one, or more objects.

(Mitias 1986: 54)

In other words, Mitias is hypothesising Hospers would argue that he, Mitias, is engaging in an essentially circular argument. But art does have a distinctive quality, continues Mitias, mainly because:

It is a *purposive*, i.e., significant form, a form capable of realizing a meaningful experience in which we are delighted, enlightened, inspired, and in which the very heart of our imagination is *enlivened*. That is, I am able to distinguish a fine work of art from an ordinary object, or artefact, by the fact that the former invites me or presents itself to my sensibility as a purposive form.[2]

(Mitias 1986: 55)

And elsewhere we find Mitias arguing that what distinguishes a fine work of art from any natural scene, for example, is that the fundamental character of the fine work of art is *human purposiveness*, so that on perceiving Renoir's *Gabrielle*:

I do not respond only actively to the complex order of aesthetic qualities which please my vision but also to the human element, to the human qualities which are pregnant, i.e., potential, in the portrait as a representation and which transcend what is immediately given. In perceiving this work, I recreate, as Dewey and Croce would say, the object in my perception and partly participate in the world in which Renoir lived when he was creating this piece.

(Mitias 1986: 56)

157

The view that art exists on the basis of unexhibited properties which transcend what is immediately given and that come to life in the aesthetic experience, is one with which, in the abstract at least, I concur. I have thus argued that our (cognitive) relations to the visual image involve unexhibited properties in the form of *life values* (our experientially derived knowledge understood in the light of our biology) and that our understanding of these relations, although primarily non-discursive, can result in cognitive transformations which lead to the image appearing to possess affective import, and so forth.

I am less certain, however, that these unexhibited properties and their effects in the general sense used by Mitias (they 'humanize' the visual image, they give it *human purposiveness*, they involve an 'enlivenment of the very heart of our imagination', etc.) are sufficient to be capable of offering objective criteria to distinguish between art and artefact. (It might be that someone possessed of a cheap reproduction, not considered by the art world to be of any artistic worth whatsoever, nonetheless appears to relate to it in terms of *human purposiveness*, as defined by Mitias.)

Mitias' view that we 'recreate' a painting in our perception thereby in part participating in our imagination in the artist's world, is to some extent shared by Wollheim when he talks about the artist's intention: 'understanding the experience of art takes the form ... of coming to see the work that causes the experience as in turn the effect of an intentional activity on the part of the artist' (1986: 8).

The intention that motivates the activity, continues Wollheim, should not be equated with the bare intention to produce a work of art, however, but must include desires, beliefs, emotions, commitments, and wishes, some of which arise from deep in the artist's psyche and some of which are unthinkable outside the history and traditions of painting. None of these factors would be influential on the way the artist works, however, if it were not for further significant beliefs held:

These are beliefs about how the resultant painting will be perceived, and the artist must believe that, when a particular intention is fulfilled in his work, then an adequately sensitive, adequately informed, spectator will tend to have experiences in front of the painting that will disclose this intention.

(Wollheim 1987: 8)

While Wollheim, like Mitias, emphasizes the unexhibited in painting and believes that it is available to the sensitive percipient, he also emphasizes the need for the artist to be aware of the potential effect a finished work will have on the percipient; this too is a necessary part of the artist's intention. In this way the artist's intention is not something that exists as a disembodied, purely mental phenomena, it is integrally tied to the artist's engagement with the medium.

This emphasis on engagement is substantiated by Collingwood (1938) when he proposes that the work of art is inseparable from the activity that brings it about so that, in the case of painting, we are necessarily talking about the development of the artist's intention through the medium of paint.[3]

Wollheim extends his views on the significance of an artist's intentions by introducing the term *thematization*, which at one point he defines as arising, 'out of the agent's [the artist's] attempt to organize an inherently inert material so that it will become serviceable for the carriage of meaning' (25).[4] (Wollheim does, however, go on to recognize the translation problem I have referred to throughout this book when he says, 'thematization by an artist must reach to aspects of painting too fine-grained for language to follow it. These will include minute aspects, and overall aspects, and relational aspects'.)

Both Mitias and Wollheim therefore stress the role the artist's intentions (which can involve desires, beliefs, emotions, etc.) play in creating the work of art and both believe that it can be partially recovered by the sensitive percipient, thereby enabling distinctions to be made between art and other phenomena. As Wollheim implies, however, the only way in which artists can hope for the percipient to engage in this process of recovery is by paying close attention to how they visually represent the world:

It must from the start be recognized that the only way in which an artist can endow an internal spectator with experiences, or, more fundamentally, with a repertoire, is through the way in which the artist depicts whatever it is – in these cases, a figure – that this spectator confronts. What the unrepresented spectator is to see, or think, or feel, must be reconstructed from how the represented figure is represented.

(Wollheim 1987: 164–6)

Wollheim's emphasis on the visual qualities in visual art is important because, as Mitias indicates, although they may not constitute an end in themselves, they are nonetheless a necessary *means to an end* (even when the artist has perhaps no clear end in mind when physically engaged in the medium). Without these qualities initially in some way holding the percipient's attention, the process of recovering an artist's intentions – the process of an image becoming 'humanized', thereby, as Mitias says, appealing to our cognitive imagination in all its diversity – would simply not occur. From this perspective we can, I believe, begin to positively examine the possibilities of what constitutes the representational visual *art* image.

The way in which the representational art image initially captures our attention is through the artist's capacity to meaningfully visually represent a subject – *whatever it may be* (regarding my emphasis, see chapter 7.9). The artist – and I am thinking in particular of accomplished painters and certain photographers because of their *control* over their medium – possesses the capacity to present us not merely with a 'snapshot' image of the phenomenal world but with one in which things visual are heightened thereby making them, in one sense, more 'real' than our typical perceptions of the world itself.

The ways in which this 'heightened perception' come about are numerous but begin with a fact that is *gratis* in that it is common to virtually all types of still visual imagery, namely, the capacity to isolate our visual perceptions from the normally intersensorially perceived phenomenal world. Thus, whatever the original sensorily involved nature of the subject, as *re*presented we are left with only its visual characteristics – and it is hardly surprising, therefore, that this should result in an initial heightening of visual perception due to a focusing of attention on these characteristics.

But this does not in itself necessarily result in the visual image constituting *art* (if it did then *any* image would obtain this status). What visual art typically possesses is the capacity to *deeply involve us* in its illusory world. This involvement can have the effect, as Berleant has proposed, that 'The viewer activates the painting, turning it from a physical object into a perceptual one and, conversely, the painting imposes itself on the viewer, forcing eye, body and thought to accommodate to its demands' (1986: 104).

There are various ways in which this process of deep involvement by initially visual means can be perpetrated. In the case of the skilful portrait favouring chiaroscuro, for example, the perci-pient is in the position of having to 'recover', probably from only a few brushstroke clues, the half of the face hidden by 'shadow'. In this way, through what can be thought of as a *cognitive effort*, the picture can assume a heightened visual (and ultimately cognitive) significance.

Landscape painting is often so constructed as to invite an almost physical involvement through a visual 'lead in' to its illusory space and time continuum.[5] For example, our perception of *The Hay-Wain* tends to begin with the left side of the nearest bank where we encounter the picture's dog. It is neither arbitrarily positioned nor posed, however, because the turn of its head directs our atten-tion 'across' the stream to the wain. Our attentions may then be drawn 'upwards' to the large expanse of sky with its billowing clouds. These are not *any* clouds but ones so artistically contrived as to suggest the quality of movement, and so forth (cf. chapter 7.2). In this (artistic) way we become deeply involved with the image's potential to engender its full existential life, the meaning suggested by its forms.

But even in works whose forms do not so obviously invite our involvement, such is the quality of their visual rendition that they often suggest a more subtle form of involvement. A still life by Char-din is not *any* picture of a table with jugs and fruit but one which, through the painter's artistic skills to render form through an expert use of colour, light and shade, almost invites our tactile ex-ploration of the picture.

It is by involving us in these and many other ways that pictures communicate an artist's intentions, intentions which, it has to be emphasized, are not communicable by any other means – they can *only* be communicated in virtue of the artist's developed *visual* understanding of the phenomenal world.

And here it also has to be emphasized that when the art theore-tician fails to fully take into account the significance of an art work's visual dimension – perhaps by referring to a general theory of art which does not properly differentiate mediums – this often results in convoluted and unsubstantiated notions about the ways in which an artist's intentions are recoverable. In such cases the theoretician typically concentrates on developing a highly abstracted, idealized, and often philosophical account of the relations between artists, their work, and public.[6]

But even confining ourselves to the initially visual effects of visual art does not mean that we are capable of *comprehensively* recovering artists' intentions – a hermeneutic dimension I have already elaborated upon at some length when referring to the views of Gombrich (see in particular 6.7). In other words, in spite of sometimes exaggerated claims, it is extremely unlikely that through the vehicle of their work artists are capable of *duplicating* in us the intentions and concomitant mental states that lead to the work in the first instance.[7]

By characterizing representational art in this way (the potential to deeply involve through the quality of its visual characteristics understood in the light of our biology and experience) I am not proposing that either art or our aesthetic response to it is contingent upon a purely sensuous appreciation of its architectonic qualities. In the final analysis, these qualities function merely as catalysts in so far as, by deeply involving us, they can direct us to our personal and experientially derived understanding of the world with all the (cognitive) ramifications I have argued this involvement implies.

This does not mean that so-called 'banal' imagery is entirely incapable of involving us, but it is typically a transitory involvement often caused by the purely sensational nature of the subject – a particularly violent image in a newspaper or a sexually explicit image in a magazine, for example.[8] However, although such imagery may be initially capable of activating some of the cognitive processes I have described, these typically remain undeveloped because of the image's (initially visual) incapacity to deeply involve us.

(It also has to be said that even when banal imagery does potentially exhibit some artistic worth – as is increasingly the case with certain photographs printed in the better newspapers and their accompanying supplements, for example – such is their scale, the ephemerality of their material constituent (paper), their (lack of) quality of reproduction, coupled with our expectations as to their worth – that they tend to instigate no more than a passing glance before we turn the page. It is possible, however, that were these images presented in their original form in a permanent and public collection to which we could return at our leisure, they would be more likely to instigate a deep and lasting involvement typically associated with *art*.)

162

8.3   AESTHETIC EXPERIENCE AS INVOLVEMENT

In this section and the next I turn to my proposal that what can appear as marked differences between certain aesthetic theories are partially explicable by viewing them as an emphasis on the different cognitive stages of the transformational processes I have described. In particular, I shall attempt to show that aspects of those theories which contend that 'distancing' from the work of art is a necessary condition for aesthetic experience, can share aspects in common with those which contend that aesthetic experience is integrally related to our involvement with art. In this section I examine the view, primarily by referring to Berleant's phenomenological approach to aesthetics, that aesthetic experience relates to our involvement.

Berleant (1986) proposes that in the modern age questions about the nature of art have tended to centre around the idea of experience, this paralleling the shift in philosophy from matters of ontology to those of epistemology. In place of starting from an examination of the nature of the universe and then to the human place in the order of things, we have come, since Descartes and Kant, to the discovery that all inquiry has its inception in the human situation. Whatever the nature of the world may be, we can only come to know it as human beings and are therefore less likely to ask what makes something *art* than we are to ask how our *experience* of art can be explained, and in this way, 'the locus of art lies not in the object but in the attitude we assume in experiencing it' (93).

There are at least three approaches that may be taken in grounding a theory of aesthetic attitude, says Berleant. The first is the philosophical-historical argument which proposes since we recognize that all experience and knowledge must rest on the human person, this is true of the particular domain we call art.[9] Thus it is the (special aesthetic) attitude we assume (as human beings) in appreciation that is the essential factor.[10] The second is psychological because, as a perceptual event the experience of art would appear to fall quite naturally within the purview of psychology and the characterization of such experience might be considered the proper province of the psychological sciences. There is, however, a third argument which Berleant favours and calls the argument from the phenomena of art.

The argument is phenomenological because it attempts to set

aside all preconceptions about what aesthetic experience must or should be. Such an argument *begins* with the occasion of such experiences and not with any philosophical encumbrances about the structure of the world or of experience itself, presumptions about human nature, or about the values sustained by art.

The other sense in which the argument is phenomenological is that it attempts to base itself on a purely descriptive mode of characterization – to rest its concepts, distinctions and theoretical shape in the actual occurrence of art and the aesthetic in *human experience* (94). Berleant develops his theme by referring to the views of Dewey:

> Dewey adopts a still more explicit recognition of total organic involvement in art. The biological, evolutionary model underlies his account of experience and, when he turns to art, he applies the same factors. Whether one's interests be scientific or aesthetic, 'the ultimate matter of both emphases in experience is ... the constant rhythm that marks the interaction of the live creature with his surroundings'. The function of art is to restore 'the union of sense, need, impulse and action characteristic of the live creature'. Such experience is integrated and consummated in what Dewey calls 'an experience', the distinguishing marks of the aesthetic.
>
> (Berleant 1986: 98–9; Dewey 1934: 15, 25)

The views of Merleau-Ponty are also referred to, particularly regarding visual art: 'Since things and my body are made of the same stuff, vision must somehow take place in them; their manifest visibility must be repeated in the body by a secret visibility' (Berleant 1986: 99; Merleau-Ponty 1964: 16).

Such accounts, continues Berleant, reflect a development that extends aesthetic experience well beyond a state of mind that is separate and distinct from the aesthetic object, beyond a psychological attitude or an act of consciousness. They join in stressing involvement, ranging from multi-sensory synaesthesia to somatic action and continuity with the object, and in this way, 'the idea of unitary perception in aesthetic experience has gradually taken form and has shaped an alternative to the disinterestedness theory' (99).

Berleant thus maintains that art and aesthetic experience can only be understood by referring to the total situation in which the objects, activities, and experiences of art occur, a situation he terms the *aesthetic field*. The aesthetic field involves the central 'elements' of: the art object, the percipient, the artist and the performer. These elements are in turn conditioned by biological, psychological, material and technological, and social and cultural factors. Using all of these elements to analyse aesthetic experience, nine principal features emerge, says Berleant. Aesthetic experience is: active-receptive, qualitative, sensuous, immediate, intuitive, non-cognitive, unique, intrinsic, and integral (1970: 97–158).

The conclusion of Berleant's argument is that certain key forces seem regularly to be present in aesthetic experience. All of these are contingent upon the recognition of the person not being a 'mind alone' but an *embodied* consciousness: 'a conscious organism or incorporated awareness who attains reflexivity and completion only in transactions with objects and events' (1986: 104). There is, then, a *participatory* engagement of perceiver and artistic object, an engagement that is not seen as being confined to the visual arts:

> Every art, painting, dance, poetry and architecture, demands to be activated in order to be realized. Whether or not a performer is required for this is less crucial a consideration than the fact that the appreciative perceiver must make his or her own contribution to transform the art object into an art work.
>
> (Berleant 1986: 105)

I have referred to Berleant's views not only because they are influential in the 'phenomenology of aesthetics' (cf. Lindauer 1981: 52) but also because, like my own, they emphasize that our relations to the world, art, and aesthetics involve the following. First, as human beings we are in the possession of an 'embodied consciousness' and this necessarily affects our perceptual and cognitive relations to the world – a perspective I have qualified from a neuropsychological perspective at length. (For example, in chapter 4.6, when developing the idea of right-hemisphere ACMs, I referred to the views of Merleau-Ponty regarding *maximum grasp* and in particular to Dreyfus' views on human consciousness. In chapter 5, I complemented the possible evolutionary origins of our embodied status, referred to in chapter 3.2, by introducing a developmental perspective, that is, by referring to how children assimilate the world through intersensorial perception and how this affects their drawing and adult picture perception.)

And then, Berleant's emphasis that our relations to art are not passive but involve *participatory engagement* (the viewer activates the painting ... the painting imposes itself on the viewer, etc.) strongly relates to my argument that, for evolutionary and biological reasons, pictures are perceived as possessing a *full existential life* to which we subsequently respond (cf. chapters 4.7, 5.5, 6.3, 6.4, 6.5, and, in particular, 7.2 and 7.3).

Berleant's conclusion that aesthetic experience is associated with nine principal features, all of which are essentially biologically and intuitively based, in turn shares aspects in common with my views on how the right hemisphere processes images (actively, directly, holistically, intuitively, intersensorially, without recourse to language, etc.).

Consequently, although Berleant does not include in his thesis any direct reference to the brain's biology and its possible effects, as I have done, like me he sees our relations to art and aesthetic experience as being materially explicable so that, 'The experience of art is neither religious nor mystical; it is eminently worldly. Not only are sensory qualities present in the immediacy of aesthetic experience; relations are often there as well' (1970: 113).

There is, however, a noticeable distinction between Berleant's views and my own on the eventual effects of our involvement with works of art. Thus while he argues at great length for the idea of a participatory engagement, he fails to take into account the possible cognitive and aesthetic effects of our *inability to respond* to this engagement, at least in relation to the representational visual image.[11] These effects, I have argued, culminate in affective import, a state associated with a psychological 'distancing' from the work of art. What begins, therefore, as an involvement in the work of art for biological, evolutionary, neuropsychologically substantiated and, in general, existentially related reasons, paradoxically culminates – in virtue of *cathectic transference* – in a necessary psychological 'distancing' from this involvement for compensatory reasons (cf. chapter 7.6). I return to Berleant's views later in this chapter.

8.4   AESTHETIC EXPERIENCE AS DISTANCE

My conclusion that a certain form of aesthetic experience I have described as affective import is associated with the percipient coming to be distanced from an art work's phenomenal connotations, although primarily developed from the neuropsychological data, shares aspects in common with more traditional theories involving the theory of disinterestedness. This theory suggests that our aesthetic relations to art involve a special attitude which considers the art object for its own sake, 'divorced', as it were, from the real world.

The theory has its origins at least as far back as Kant (1790, 1914) and its more recent exponents include Bell (1914), Langer (1967), Osborne (1970), Hospers (1976), and Stolnitz (1960, 1986). Although such theories often differ in their emphases (cf. Dziemidok 1986: 144–5) they share fundamental aspects in common, as Hospers suggests:

It must suffice to say that there is one kind of *attitude* which is fundamental to all of the experiences described, and without which the use of the term 'esthetic' to apply to anything distinctive in our experience must quite disappear. This fundamental attitude consists in the separation of the esthetic experience from the needs and desires of everyday life and from the responses which we customarily make to our environment as practical human beings.

(Hospers 1976: 4)

Undoubtedly, however, the most influential, most quoted and widely accepted version of the theory (Crossley 1975) is Edward Bullough's concept of 'psychical distance' (1912) and it is the one that I shall examine here.[12] Bullough introduces his concept by asking us to:

Imagine a fog at sea: for most people it is an experience of acute unpleasantness ... it is apt to produce feelings of peculiar anxiety, fears of invisible dangers, strains of watching and listening for unlocalised signals ... Nevertheless, a fog at sea can be the source of intense relish and enjoyment. Abstract from the experience of the sea fog, for the moment, its danger and practical unpleasantness ... direct the attention to the features 'objectively' constituting the phenomenon – the veil surrounding you with an opaqueness as of transparent milk, blurring the outlines of things and distorting their shapes into weird grotesqueness ... note the curious creamy smoothness of the water, hypocritically denying as it were any suggestion of danger; and, above all, the strange solitude and remoteness from the world, as it can be found on only the highest mountain tops: and the experience may acquire, in its uncanny mingling of repose and terror, a flavour of such concentrated poignancy and delight as to contrast sharply with the blind and tempered anxiety of its other aspects. This contrast, often emerging with startling suddenness, is like a momentary switching on of some new current, or the passing ray of a brighter light, illuminating the outlook upon perhaps the most ordinary and familiar objects – an impression which we experience sometimes in instants of direst extremity, when our practical interest snaps like a wire from sheer over-tension, and we watch the consummation of some impending catastrophe with the marvelling unconcern of a mere spectator.

(Bullough 1983: 58–60)

Psychical distance is essentially a difference of outlook due to the insertion of Distance (a specific mental state) which appears to lie 'between our own self and its affections' so that, as in the fog, 'the transformation by Distance is produced in the first instance by putting the phenomenon, so to speak, out of gear with our practical, actual self; by allowing it to stand outside the context of our personal needs and ends – in short by looking at it "objectively"' (60–1).

The working of Distance is not simple, however, because it involves both a *negative* inhibitory aspect – the cutting-out of the practical side of things and our practical attitude to them – and a *positive* side – the elaboration of the experience on the new basis created by the inhibitory action of Distance (61).

But the insertion of Distance does not imply an impersonal, purely intellectual relation to phenomena – on the contrary it is often highly emotionally coloured and of a peculiar character in that, 'Its peculiarity lies in that the personal character of the relation has been, so to speak, filtered. It has been cleared of the practical, concrete nature of its appeal, without, however, thereby losing its original constitution' (65). Distance is also variable both in accordance with the distancing power of the individual and the character of the object perceived. There are two ways of losing distance: either to 'under-distance' or to 'over-distance' – i.e. when the percipient of an art work becomes either too involved (thereby not properly distinguishing between 'art' and 'life') or too remote from it (in which case the work lacks personal significance).

Maximal distance does not, therefore, create the best conditions for aesthetic experience to occur. In fact, optimal conditions are met when the 'the distance is smallest but still present' (this is the essence of Bullough's principle of the 'antinomy of distance', see 67–8, for example).

Distinct art forms, in virtue of their respective communicative natures, coupled with their manner of presentation, are more likely to under- or over-distance. Theatre and dance in particular tend towards an under-distancing because of the presence of living human beings as communicative vehicles for the art form. Next comes sculpture, because 'Though not using a living bodily medium, yet the human form in its full spatial materiality constitutes a similar threat to Distance' (79). Paintings are less likely to under-distance because they possess:

> intrinsically a much greater Distance – because neither their space (perspective and imaginary space) nor their lighting coincides with our (actual) space or light, and the usual reduction in scale of the represented objects prevents a feeling of undue proximity. Besides, painting always retains to some extent a *two*-dimensional character, and this character supplies *eo ipso* a Distance.
>
> (Bullough 1983: 96)

Bullough also includes in his theory the respective distancing powers of music and architecture which as the 'two most abstract of all arts show a remarkable fluctuation in their Distances' (80).

Bullough's theory of 'psychical distance' is not, then, confined to the visual arts just as it is not easily confined to either philosophical or psychological aesthetics. Exactly where the theory is placed in the history of aesthetics is less important, however, than its lasting influence. Nonetheless, at first sight it might appear that the theory, with its emphasis on the work of art being separated from the needs and desires of everyday life, shares little in common with my own with its initial emphasis on the importance of our experientially derived relations to the work of art.

In his 'fog at sea' analogy and the subsequent logic of his reasoning, however, Bullough by no means disregards the effects of the experiential on our eventual aesthetic relations to art. We thus find him implying that the traveller is initially apt to experience acute unpleasantness for purely practical reasons – for example, the possibility of shipwreck as implied by 'strains of watching and listening for unlocalised signals'. It is only *after* this 'practical side of things and our practical attitude to them' has been 'cut-out' through the negative and *inhibitory* action of Distance that (aesthetic) experience can be (positively) elaborated upon.

In this way, Bullough logically (if paradoxically) implies that aesthetic experience and its elaboration is integrally related to the existential in the sense that it is only through a *suppression* of the practical through the inhibitory action of Distance that an object comes to be aesthetically perceived. Aesthetic perception is therefore generated in virtue of its contrast not to *any* perception but one firmly rooted in our experientially derived understanding of the phenomenal world, and it is this contrast that makes aesthetic experience in some way *special*.

Bullough's emphasis on the suppressive or inhibitory working of Distance and its consequent aesthetic connotations therefore shares aspects in common with the suppressive/adaptive workings of my *cathectic transference* process which occurs because of our *inability to respond* to our experientially derived understanding of an image's existential life (cf. chapter 7.5).[13]

Bullough elaborates the nature of Distancing by implying that it comes about through transformational processes which, as I have proposed regarding the transformational processes that lead to affective import, have *specific* points of transition from the practical to the 'psychic'. We thus saw:

> This contrast, often emerging with startling suddenness, is like a momentary switching on of some new current, or the passing of a brighter light, illuminating the outlook upon perhaps the most ordinary and familiar objects – an impression which we experience sometimes in instants of direst extremity, when our practical interest snaps like a wire from sheer over-tension.
>
> (Bullough 1983: 60)

This transition from a practical to a potentially aesthetic mental state is therefore 'startlingly sudden'; it is a point which can be compared to the 'momentary switching on of some new current, or the passing of a brighter light'; it can be compared to the 'snapping of a wire' – these allusions implying a particular and significant point of transition between one mental state and another.

Bullough's view that the effects of Distancing can result in aesthetic experience also shares aspects in common with my own regarding the effects of cathectic transference which can result in affective import. I have thus proposed that cathectic transference can result (for vicarious reasons) in a mental state associated with the percipient becoming psychologically estranged from the existential component of the work of art, this leading to the primarily visual nature of the work assuming an extraordinary significance ('It is as if the normally intersensorially perceived phenomenal world in all its variety, complexity and implications has become concentrated into a "visually encapsulated island", that is, one in which only things visual assume import', etc. Chapter 7.6).

Bullough implies a similar 'funnelling' of emotional response (due to a suppression of existentially derived tendencies) from the 'real' to the 'psychological' (with consequent extraordinary psychological and perceptual effects) when he says, regarding the effects of Distance, that: 'Its peculiarity lies in that the personal character of the relation has been, so to speak, *filtered*. It has been cleared of the practical, concrete nature of its appeal, without, however, thereby losing its original constitution' (my emphasis).

8.5 THE RELATIVE AESTHETIC

In these last two sections we have seen two contrasting yet influential views on aesthetic response as represented by the theories of Berleant and Bullough. Thus, central to Berleant's argument is that aesthetic response is contingent upon our involvement (participatory engagement) with the work of art, whereas central to Bullough's is that aesthetic response is contingent upon a wilful 'psychical distancing' from too great an involvement. I have attempted to show that the views of both Berleant and Bullough share aspects in common with my own.

Berleant thus argues, as I have done, that our relations to art and aesthetic experience are contingent upon our embodied status, that they involve participatory engagement which does not involve an act of consciousness (the wilful adoption of a certain mental attitude), that they are primarily intuitive, and so forth. His views differ from mine, however, in their failure to take into account the aesthetic effects of our *inability to respond* to works of art, at least regarding the representational visual image.

Bullough's views share aspects in common with my own in their emphasis that our aesthetic relations to art involve a *suppression* of our normal engagement with the phenomenal world; that this suppression has specific points of transition, and that the (transformational) effects of this suppression can result in the work of art appearing to become 'distanced' from (existential) reality. Unlike my views, however, Bullough argues that Distance is contingent upon the wilful adoption of a certain mental attitude (whereas I have argued that this suppressive process is automatic).

The question now arises as to which aesthetic theory are we to believe in – the one proposed by Berleant, which regards aesthetic experience as being integrally related to our existentially associated involvement with the work of art – the one proposed by Bullough, which regards aesthetic experience as being integrally related to a calculated suppression of this involvement – or the one I have proposed, which regards aesthetic experience as being integrally related to both our involvement *and* its (psychological) suppression for essentially compensatory and adaptive reasons.

To properly answer this question it has to be fully recognized that different art forms are psychologically distinct in virtue of the respective communicative distinctions inherent in their medium forms, and that these distinctions typically produce quite different response tendencies in the percipient. We do not respond to a piece of music in the same way that we respond to either a painting or a piece of theatre. As I proposed in the opening section of my introduction to this book: our relations to individual art forms suppose distinct *ways of knowing* so that the one pertaining to the visual arts can be distinguished from the one pertaining to literature, music, or any of the other arts. This has as a possible corollary that aspects of our mental life are specialized and that different ways of knowing are neither necessarily compatible nor inter-translatable, etc.

From this it follows that different art forms are likely to involve us in different ways and by different degrees. In their respective emphases the theories of Berleant and Bullough are not necessarily 'wrong', therefore, in that both may have implications for certain art forms but less so for others – just as my own theory has specific implications for the way of knowing relevant to the form associated with the representational visual image. In other words, different art forms generate distinct modes of aesthetic response which should not be confused, one with the other.

It is unlikely, however, that either aesthetician would agree to their theories being so confined, in that both profess to have constructed a *general* theory of aesthetic response, that is, one which applies equally to *all* major art forms. In this way, both aestheticians presume that all art forms share, or should share, a *common way of knowing*, with the implication that they share a common aesthetic. This presumption means, however, that the respective theories inevitably run into difficulties.

Bullough's theory, for example, initially takes into account the different communicative natures of distinct art forms and the consequent potential aesthetic effects of these differences. Distinct mediums are prone to fluctuation in their tendency to under- or over-distance, that is, in their tendency to more or less involve us (and therefore to more or less create the optimum aesthetic experience). However, because Bullough is intent on constructing a *general* theory of aesthetic response, he proposes that this tendency towards extremes is aesthetically undesirable. It is a tendency which can be compensated for, however, by the 'distancing power of the individual', that is, by the percipient wilfully adopting the 'correct' mental attitude towards the art form in question.

In this way Bullough attempts to rescue his theory from an obvious difficulty – mainly the simple fact that different art forms, in virtue of their distinct communicative modes, *do* elicit different kinds and degrees of response in the individual, responses that cannot be readily equated.

My criticism of Bullough's views apply equally to those of Berleant. Thus Berleant's emphasis on participatory engagement with a consequent kind of aesthetic experience, may very well apply to certain contemporary art forms, as he readily points out, 'The contemporary arts in particular frequently insist on experiences of engagement by provoking us into movement or action or by forcing us into adjustments in vision and imagination' (1986: 96). This does not mean, however, that we can successfully participate in all art forms, as I have pointed out regarding the more traditional art form of representational painting (although Berleant would probably disagree).[14]

And surely the whole attraction of distinct art forms lies in their individual capacities to communicate differently, thereby involving us by different degrees and in different ways. Why, then, should we expect different art forms to elicit a *common* aesthetic response any more than we expect artists gifted in certain media to be equally gifted in others?

This essentially *relative* approach to aesthetic response applies equally to particular forms within art forms, representational as distinct from abstract painting, for example. Thus, because my theory applies to the representational visual image does not mean that it automatically applies to abstract painting just because it so happens that both forms are associated with the visual arts. That is, because both forms initially visually communicate their meaning does not mean that they communicate in the same way or possess similar aesthetic potentials.

In neuropsychological terms, because both forms are initially processed through the visual system, does not indicate that they are similarly *cognized*, that they elicit similar *ways of knowing*. This does not mean that either visual form is more or less potentially aesthetically significant – in the same way it does not mean that the aesthetic potential inherent in distinct art forms is more or less aesthetically significant. The implication is, however, that the nature of aesthetic response generated by distinct art forms simply differs; in other words, aesthetic response is a relative phenomenon contingent upon distinct laws of transformation.

Chapter Nine

THE TRANSFORMATIONAL PLANES

9.1 INTRODUCTION

My theory of aesthetic response centres around the view that, for neuropsychological and evolutionary reasons, our initially visual perceptions of the representational visual image can cause a complex series of cognitive transformations which result in a special kind of experience.

In this, my concluding chapter, I formalize these transformations by dividing them into ten hypothetical stages which I have termed planes. These are meant to describe distinct mental processes and should not be confused with the visual representation's either material or optically constituted planes – its two-dimensional plane or the (illusory) three-dimensional planes certain marks on this surface may produce, for example.

The planes, which are meant to show a development beginning with our dominantly right-hemisphere and concluding with our dominantly left-hemisphere associated perceptions of the representational image, are described as follows. The surface plane, the three-dimensional plane, the representational plane, the content plane, the existential plane, the paradoxical plane, the response plane, the affective plane, the aesthetic plane, and the discursive plane.

9.2 THE SURFACE PLANE

The surface plane describes the process concerned with the purely optical registration of light falling on our retinas providing the bases for sensations of light and colour (brightness, hue, and saturation). These sensations subsequently inform how the two-dimensional surface is spatially arranged and divided. For example, the registration of two or more contrasting hue and/or tonal values (depending on whether colour is involved) may indicate the existence of certain patterns and/or different shapes occupying separate locations on the surface.[1]

At this primary stage in our perceptions, an image's visual elements are registered in a purely mechanical (automatic) fashion which can be compared to how light is registered on a film after passing through a camera lens.

9.3   THE THREE-DIMENSIONAL PLANE

The three-dimensional plane describes that process whereby our registration of the surface plane's visual elements provides the optical system with sufficient units of information to enable conclusions to be drawn regarding their three-dimensional character. That is, whether they constitute planes, volumes and distances within an illusory perspectival space.

Included in this process is the search for whether certain forms have principal or branching axes, this search being derived from and corresponding to the way in which it has been argued that the brain processes visual-spatial information derived from the phenomenal world (cf. 3.3). The search is therefore governed by attempts to 'compute' a generalized, three-dimensional view of certain visual elements arranged on a two-dimensional surface.

Any conclusions drawn regarding an image form's three-dimensionality necessarily remain hypothetical, however, because of its materially two-dimensional nature. For example, whereas a particular arrangement of visual elements may optically suggest the solid and three-dimensional existence of a cube or sphere, this perception cannot be confirmed or refuted as it could be in the phenomenal world (by an alteration of our perspective point, tactile examination, etc.).[2]

This (mental) reconstitution of certain visual elements into three-dimensional spatial relations and forms is also an automatic process and does not, therefore, need to be learned (cf. 3.3, 3.6, 4.7, 6.2, and 7.2.).

9.4   THE REPRESENTATIONAL PLANE

The representational plane, which describes those mental processes activated by conclusions drawn from the three-dimensional plane, is catalytic in the sense that it draws from our visually encapsulated knowledge of the phenomenal world stored in memory (cf. 4.2–7).

Such is the nature of certain image forms that they are perceived as sharing visual-spatial characteristics in common with those which typically define the nature of form in the phenomenal world. There exists, therefore, a direct visual-spatial correspondence between image forms and their phenomenal referents. For example, such is the visual-spatial nature of certain image forms in *The Hay-Wain* that their appearance corresponds to those typically defined as trees, clouds, streams, and so forth (cf. 6.2 and 7.2.).

Although the representational plane is more (cognitively) complex than the surface and three-dimensional planes (because it draws from visually encapsulated knowledge stored in memory), it too is a primarily automatic process not requiring learning.

However, this does not imply that a familiarity with the specific visual-spatial characteristics of an image form's referents is not acquired through life experience – this logically has to be the case in order for an image form to *re*present something extant in the phenomenal world.[3]

The operations of the representational plane are therefore effective not only because of the activation of certain innately determined processes (the capacity to see in a certain way) but also because of their relations to experientially derived information stored in memory. At this stage in the transformation process, then, an empirical as distinct from a purely nativistic paradigm begins to play its part in our perceptions of the representational visual image.

9.5   THE CONTENT PLANE

The content plane describes those mental processes concerned with establishing the *collective* visual identity of the individual spatial relations and forms identified by the representational plane process. As is true of the representational plane, the successful operation of the content plane requires reference to visually encapsulated knowledge stored in memory. For example, the collective identity of the individual image forms: trees, clouds, streams, and so forth, when juxtaposed in a manner relevant to our experientially derived knowledge, denotes the visual equivalent for what is typically described as a 'landscape'; other collective image forms may denote a 'still life', a 'portrait', and so forth.[4]

This facility to relate illusory spatial relations and forms to our holistic, visually encapsulated (life) experience of their referents, affords the representational image an homogeneity and credibility for a number of interrelated reasons.

For example, once we have established the holistic visual identity of an image (and this typically occurs at a glance), we are in a better position to clarify any ambiguities implied by its individual spatial relations and forms. Thus, our holistic understanding of *The Hay-Wain* as a 'landscape' leads us to expect that its individual image forms should occupy approximately the same relative positions, magnitudes, and so forth, as their referents when viewed from a certain perspective point. In this way, on perceiving *The Hay-Wain*, we do not conclude that some of its trees are smaller than others because they are literally represented as such. Our experientially derived visual knowledge of 'trees in a landscape' leads us to conclude that certain of the picture's trees are not smaller but simply more distant than those represented in its foreground.

Relatedly, our experientially derived understanding of the visual nature of the phenomenal world enables us to mentally substitute (in a sense 'fill in') for those parts of an image either only hinted at in a picture or else occluded by other forms. In this way, we do not conclude that that part of the stream in *The Hay-Wain* occluded by the wain itself is non-existent any more than we believe that the half of a face not seen in a portrait that favours chiaroscuro is non-existent (cf. chapters 5.5 and 8.2.).

9.6 THE EXISTENTIAL PLANE

The essential function performed by *the existential plane* process is to afford the representational image its *full existential life* thereby removing it from a purely visually encapsulated level of understanding. This process is effected by the representational image automatically releasing originally intersensorially perceived (as distinct from purely visually perceived) knowledge relevant to its phenomenal referents.[5] This information is subsequently applied to the various image forms constituting the representational image as a whole thereby adding to its credibility as a *re*presentation of the world.

For example, our originally intersensorially perceived knowledge that streams are liquid and that liquids do not resist solids, in combination with our knowledge that cart-wheels are solid, circular and of an approximate dimension, enables us to conclude that *The Hay-Wain*'s wain-wheels are partially *submerged*; that its stream must be little more than ankle deep, and so forth.

It is thus generally the case that the existential life of any one representational visual image is as comprehensive as our (intersensorially perceived) understanding of its referent's character traits and how these might interact in the phenomenal world. It is this understanding which affords us a *maximum grasp* of the representational visual image (cf. chapters 4.6, 5.5, and 7.2.).

9.7   THE PARADOXICAL PLANE

The paradoxical plane describes that stage in the transformational process whose operations were detailed in my *paradox of perceptual belief hypothesis* (cf. 7.2); that is, it describes that mental state which arises from two potentially conflicting belief systems activated by our perceptions of the representational visual image. Thus, if the representational image assumes a full existential life because of its capacity to activate the several mental processes or planes so far described, this perception has to be contrasted with our (better) knowledge that this life is necessarily as illusory as the image forms which constitute it.

Therefore, in virtue of their capacity to *re*present, certain marks on a two-dimensional surface come to psychologically suggest our complex, experientially derived understanding of the phenomenal world and yet, because of their two-dimensionality, they necessarily remain distinctly apart from it. In this way the representational visual image comes to exist in an *equivocal reality*. That is, a psychologized existential reality which, once activated, persists even when information from the same (representational) source and inputted through the same (visual) modality simultaneously contradicts its existence.

The reason for the (psychological) persistence of equivocal reality is because the same right-hemisphere associated paradigm which evolved to enable us to instantly draw conclusions from our visual-spatial perceptions of the phenomenal world is automatically activated by its (analogic) representation, the picture itself. In spite of our understanding that the visual-spatial and existential life of a representation is merely illusory, therefore, this is insufficient to negate the sustaining effects of certain innately determined or biologically 'hardwired' responses which it activates as a special class of symbol form (cf. chapters 4.6 and 4.7).

9.8   THE RESPONSE PLANE

The response plane describes that mental stage in the transformational process where, because of the representational image's capacity to activate complex, primarily non-discursive but existentially derived information relevant to life values, it elicits certain expectations and response tendencies. For example, it could be the case that our perception of the cloud formation in *The Hay-Wain* suggests a potential for movement, or that erotic imagery activates certain sexual expectations and responses.

Such expectations and possible responses are subsequently 'interrupted' (in a sense, contradicted), however, by our understanding that they cannot 'complete' (be resolved) in terms of their activating stimuli, the representational image itself, because of its materially constrained (illusory) nature.

In this way, after having activated certain expectations and response tendencies, the representational visual image subsequently comes to be perceived as existentially deficient. This perception does not result in the (cognitive) negation of the expectations and response tendencies activated by the representation's existential life, however, because, in character with the paradoxical plane, they are sustained by the effects of innately determined mental processes initially activated by our visual perceptions.

The operations of the response plane therefore compound the essentially dissonant mental state associated with the paradoxical plane. Consequently, at this stage in the transformational process, not only does the representational image continue to be perceived as possessing an existential life but this perception can produce definite expectations and response tendencies (cf. chapters 7.3 and 7.4).

9.9   THE AFFECTIVE PLANE

The affective plane describes the essentially compensatory mental process which, in virtue of *cathectic transference*, results in the representational image appearing to possess affective import. Thus, an image's capacity to elicit expectations and response tendencies related to life values means that these (a) continue to be 'interrupted' and (b) that forms of 'completion' (resolution) are continually sought. Because completion cannot be effected by the representational image due to its materially constrained nature, however, a 'response substitution' strategy becomes activated.

However, because a successful response substitution is typically impossible, this can result in states of emotional arousal and concomitant tensions which, because of the sustaining nature of the paradoxical plane, continue for the duration of our perception of an image's full existential life.

Eventually, however, it is the representational image itself which (paradoxically) offers a form of emotional release; a way of (vicariously) completing the emotional tensions it activates. That is, with all forms of emotional belief 'blocked', the release has to be effected through some form of paradigm shift, some form of psychological change on our part. This is effected by a concentrated projection or a *cathectic transference* of the emotional tensions 'into' the one outlet readily available to perception, the representational image itself.

Such is the nature of this transference that it has the subsequent effect of transforming the representation (in the eye of the beholder) into appearing to become 'psychologically energized', into appearing to possess *affective import*.

As an essentially compensatory and adaptive mental state, affective import is associated with the tendency towards a detached exploration of an image's visual properties. Thus the image, once possessed of a full existential life, now necessarily appears strangely distanced or disembodied from it, a state that may be compared to dream perception (cf. 7.5, 7.6 and 8.4.).

9.10   THE AESTHETIC PLANE

The aesthetic plane describes that mental stage in the transformational process where the left-hemisphere associated language centres experience the effects of dominantly right-hemisphere associated perceptions and cognitions of the representational visual image. Consequently, although the mental processes that result in the representational image appearing to possess affective import are dominantly right-hemisphere generated, their effect (and affect) spreads in holistic (mental aura) form, via the brain's major and subsidiary communication pathways, to the left-hemisphere language centres.

Because this is an habitual process repeatedly induced by our perceptions of certain images, this results in the characterization of a certain kind of experience as aesthetic. Because the language centres possess no direct knowledge of the causes of this experience (thereby making it difficult to linguistically introspect), this often results in the view that it is an elusive and enigmatic phenomenon (cf. 7.7 and 8.2).

9.11 THE DISCURSIVE PLANE

The discursive plane describes those left-hemisphere generated processes which sometimes attempt to compensate for, in virtue of a *secondary level of cathectic transference*, the continuing effects of aesthetic experience. Thus, aesthetic experience is typically sustained by its role as a (vicarious) outlet for emotional tensions repeatedly induced by the effects of our dominantly right-hemisphere associated perceptions of the representational image. Such is the nature of this experience (it is enigmatic, it is different to ordinary experience, etc.), that it prompts comment in keeping with the language centre's biologically evolved tendency to conceptualize and rationalize information.

The art theoretician is, however, faced with the dilemma centred around inferring from insufficient units of information. A unit is possessed which informs of the (holistic) existence of aesthetic experience and a unit which informs that this is causally related to the object of aesthetic experience, the image itself. What is not possessed are those vital units of information relevant to the causes of aesthetic experience because of their non-discursive, right-hemisphere associated origin.

The theoretician therefore often attempts to resolve this problem by putting into effect a *secondary level of cathectic transference*. Thus, with access to vital units of information relevant to the nature of aesthetic experience 'blocked' from (discursive) consciousness, but continually motivated by their (extraordinary) psychological effect, the theoretician is in the position of having to re-channel energies. This re-channelling can result in seeing how the representational visual image, as the object of aesthetic experience, can be discursively accommodated or *talked about*.

When referred to by the percipient, the results of this strategy (the linguistically communicated message) can result in a paradigm shift. That is, a shift of attention *away* from the percipient's right-hemisphere (direct, intuitive, recognitory, etc.) and towards a left-hemisphere (indirect, discursive, recall, etc.) way of knowing the representational visual image (cf. chapter 7.8).

PSYCHOANALYSIS AND ART

INTRODUCTION

This appendix distinguishes between my theory of aesthetic response and Peter Fuller's hypothesis concerned with establishing the nature and origins of artistic creativity. Part of my need to distinguish arises because, whereas our views mutually emphasize the importance evolution and biology play in our appreciation of art, Fuller finds it necessary to substantiate his hypothesis by referring to psychoanalytic theory.[1] This results in a misconception of how we understand the representational visual image and the potentially aesthetic role it plays in our psychology and the history of art in general. Citing Fuller's views necessarily means outlining the research of the psychiatrist and paediatrician Donald Winnicott, because, as Fuller freely acknowledges, his own hypothesis draws heavily upon Winnicott's theory of culture and creative living.

DONALD WINNICOTT'S THEORY OF CULTURE AND CREATIVE LIVING

For Winnicott, the roots of all cultural activity can be traced to 'potential space', a hypothetical area which in the first year of the infant's life comes to exist between infant and mother. As an intermediate area, potential space is contrasted with the 'inner' world of the infant and the external reality which has its own dimensions and can be objectively studied.

To begin with, the infant is insufficiently cognizant to be capable of distinguishing its own being from that of the mother or part-mother and even less so from the broader environment. It is initially in the infant's interest that the mother perpetuates this illusion because it directly contributes to its potential capacity to

184

create. Winnicott thus proposes:

> The mother's adaption to the infant's needs, when good
> enough, gives the infant the *illusion* that there is an external
> reality that corresponds to the infant's own capacity to create.
> In other words, there is an overlap between what the mother
> supplies and what the child might legitimately conceive of.
>
> (Winnicott 1971: 12)

We are given an example of the mother appearing to offer her breast at exactly the same time as the infant desires it, thereby indicating that the external reality of the breast is its own creation; that is, from the infant's (cognitive) point of view, the breast appears to magically manifest itself as a result of its imagining prompted by need. It therefore believes it to be a personal creation under its omnipotent control. Because this response is habitual, the breast is, 'created by the infant over and over again out of the infant's capacity to love or (one might say) out of need' (11).

In the natural course of the infant's maturation, however, the mother's adaption lessens according to the infant's growing ability to account for the failure of adaption and to tolerate the results of frustration. For example, the infant comes to realize that the breast does not always appear at exactly the same moment it imagines it. If all goes well, the infant gains from its frustration since incomplete adaption makes objects real, that is, capable of being hated as well as loved. And here, with what Winnicott calls the gradual disillusionment of the infant, which develops from its growing awareness of a reality external to itself, we arrive at Winnicott's concepts of potential space and the transitional object. These, together with his descriptions of the early infant-mother relationship, form the basis of his theory of culture and creative living.

As the infant becomes increasingly aware of the autonomy of external reality, beginning with an awareness of its mother as an entity distinct from itself, it begins to separate the 'not-me' from the 'me'. In order for this process to succeed, however, the child requires a 'safe' area where, mainly through play, it can develop the use of symbols that stand at one and the same time for external world phenomena and phenomena being looked at. Winnicott defines this third area, which is distinct from inner and outer reality, as potential space:

> The hypothetical area that exists (but cannot exist) between

the baby and the object (mother or part mother) during the
phase of repudiation of the object as not-me, that is at the
end of being merged in with the object.

(Winnicott 1971: 107)

Potential space is therefore an intermediate area of experience
to which inner reality and external life both contribute; an area
between the subjective and what is objectively perceived.

Having begun to realize that the world is no longer under its
omnipotent control – it can no longer be imagined into being –
the infant feels a loss of omnipotence. Consequently, with the help
of good mother care, it effectively wills into being an intermediate
area of experience by way of compensation for this loss. The area
serves a dualistic function – it facilitates the separation process (sof-
tens the trauma which occurs on the realization of an external
'not-me' reality) – and yet at the same time provides an area where
ultimate separation and reality acceptance can be avoided;
avoided, because the child fills in potential space with symbolic play
and, proposes Winnicott, with all that eventually adds up to cultural life.

Creative living and cultural life, whatever its manifestation,
therefore occurs at least partially as a result of the infant's incapacity to fully come to terms with separation and reality acceptance.
Culture is, then, partially symptomatic of substitutive behaviour
resultant upon failure to accept what is termed the Reality Principle. And it is made quite clear that this behaviour continues into
adulthood, because:

It is assumed here that the task of reality acceptance is never
completed, that no human being is free from the strain of
relating inner and outer reality, and that relief from this
strain is provided by an intermediate area of experience ...
which is not challenged (arts, religion, etc.). This intermediate area is in direct continuity with the play area of the small
child who is 'lost' in play.

(Winnicott 1971: 13)

In the play area provided by potential space we find the transitional object, which, as the child's first 'not-me' possession, can be
virtually anything – a piece of blanket, a teddy bear, a rag – because
what is important is its material function as a dualistic symbol which
can be located:

186

at the place in space and time where and when the mother is in transition from being (in the baby's mind) merged with the infant and alternatively being experienced as an object to be perceived rather than conceived of. The use of an object symbolizes the union of two now separate things, baby and mother, *at the point in space and time of the initiation of their state of separateness*.

(Winnicott 1971: 96–7)

Consequently, like potential space, the transitional object presents us with a paradox because, although it is recognized as the first not-me object, one of its essential functions is to reject external reality, that is, by symbolically representing the *re*union of infant and mother. And here it should be emphasized that Winnicott is referring to the normal healthy infant with a caring mother, not to the infant deprived of adequate mother care. The play which comes about in potential space is universal, says Winnicott, and belongs to health, even though it might be that not all children are equally fortunate:

One baby is given sensitive management here where the mother is separating out from the baby so that the area of play is immense; and the next baby has so poor an experience at this phase of his or her development that there is but little opportunity for development except in terms of introversion or extroversion.

(Winnicott 1971: 108)

The quality of adult creativity, then, largely depends on infantile play whose successful realization is contingent upon adequate potential space provided by good mother care. Nurture therefore figures strongly in Winnicott's theory of culture because, 'The special feature of this place where play and cultural experience have a position is that *it depends for its existence on living experiences*, not on inherited tendencies' (108). Winnicott emphasizes, however, that his theory of culture and creative living is a very general one:

I am hoping that the reader will accept a general reference to creativity, not letting the word get lost in the successful or acclaimed creation but keeping it to the meaning that refers to a colouring of the whole attitude to external reality.

(Winnicott 1971: 65)

And elsewhere Winnicott emphasizes that the creativity which concerns him is universal; it belongs to being alive and it is necessary to separate the idea of creation from the work of art. In fact, in the final analysis it is indicated that just about anything can be creative because, 'The creativity we are studying belongs to the approach of the individual to external reality' (68). And even when referring to specific creations their range is so wide as to lose personal significance, 'It is true that a creation can be a picture or a house or a garden or a symphony or a sculpture; anything from a meal cooked at home' (67).

I return to the implications of Winnicott's theory later because now I shall introduce Peter Fuller's adaption and application of it as found in *The Naked Artist* (1983a) and *Aesthetics After Modernism* (1983b).

NEOTENY AS AN EXPLANATION FOR POTENTIAL SPACE

Fuller attempts to complement and substantiate Winnicott's theory of culture and creative living, with its emphasis on living experience, by drawing from prehistory and biology:

> Now I think we can begin to understand this problem of the biological roots of culture if we consider two quite different kinds of evidence: firstly the evidence from the study of prehistory and biological theory; and secondly that produced by recent psychoanalytic research.

> (Fuller 1983a: 12)

Drawing from the concept of potential space, Fuller informs us that culture is an outgrowth of our capacity for labile symbolization and ability to detach symbols from ourselves into a third area of experiencing which is neither quite 'objective' nor 'subjective'. It is also a comparatively recent development in the natural history of our species, having begun with Neanderthal man who, with his burial rites, simple carving incorporating bodily and sexual symbolism, and his representations of animals in painting, showed the first glimmerings of higher culture. As Neanderthal gave way to Cromagnon man, our species became increasingly culturally adept and artistically sophisticated and mainly, it is proposed, because of the important phenomena of *neoteny*.

Neoteny is the process through which the early stages and fea-

tures in the development of an animal are retained into later periods of growth, or, as Fuller puts it, it is easiest to think of it as a
sort of slowing down of growing up. Some of the features of neoteny
as found in our species are pointed out: our growth period takes
roughly twice as long as for African apes, twenty as opposed to ten
or eleven years; our comparative hairlessness, and so forth. In fact,
proposes Fuller, the well-researched differences between hairy,
squat, ape-like early Neanderthals and their Cromagnon succes-
sors, can largely be explained through neoteny.

Neoteny developed because, as our brain size increased through
evolutionary processes, a problem arose with childbirth. Fuller
thus relates how the Neanderthal's brain size was larger than
today's average; Neanderthal mothers' pelvic size, however, was
much the same as the modern adult. Neanderthal mothers must
have therefore experienced great difficulty in giving birth to infants whose skulls were too rigid to squash; the infant mortality
rate must have been as high as 90 per cent. Consequently, those
infants with a low birth to adult brain size percentage survived to
become the parents of the next generation until we reach the present when the infant's brain at birth is only 23 per cent of its
potential size.

Neoteny also led to the infant skull bones ossifying more slowly,
thereby in turn allowing a squashing of the skull which gave the
big-brained a 'new lease of birth'. (However, no attempt is made
to establish the possible significance of the relationship between
brain and skull size. Neither is mention made of exactly how neoteny led to attenuated ossification of the skull.) The relevance of
neoteny to cultural development, explains Fuller, is that so slow
did the new-born infant's growth pattern become for a greater part
in its life than ever before in higher primate history, that its relations to the world of necessity had to be mediated through the
person of the mother. In this way we very quickly arrive at Winnicott's theory of culture and creative living with its emphasis on
the importance of the infant-mother relationship. In effect, neoteny, which helped change the Neanderthal into the Cromagnon,
is the phylogenetic seat and biological cause of Winnicott's concept
of potential space and therefore creative living. Fuller can thus propose:

> Now it seems to me that we have here ... an explanation of
> why the acceleration of the biological process of neoteny in

late Neanderthal times was associated with the emergence in
our species of symbolism, art and culture. Winnicott demon-
strates that the psychological processes of the human infant –
given its strange position of absolute independence and of
absolute dependence – differs from those of other creatures.

(Fuller 1983a: 16–17)

As we saw in relation to Winnicott's theory, the infant's 'strange
position' leads to culture because, as adults are never free from the
strain of relating inner to outer reality, we continually long to imaginatively create the world. Nonetheless, continues Fuller, although
neoteny enriched our psychological processes, endowed us with the
capacity for symbolic and imaginative thought, and gave rise to a
dream life fuller than other species, it did not in itself render the
production of art possible. The roots of expression in the plastic
arts lie not only in the aesthetic instincts but also in bodily expression, and more particularly facial expression. In fact, facial
expression was probably initially the most basic and important form
of communication in our species because it helped to cement the
infant-mother social bond so necessary for the survival of the infant.

Therefore, as Winnicott has shown, continues Fuller, the
mother's face, together with her breasts, enter deeply into the
child's conception of self and other. Nonetheless, the extension of
expression from inter-somatic communication to the capacity to
create autonomous, expressive works of art, also required the evolution of the human hand which occurred simultaneously with that
of the brain and the onset of neotenous phenomena. Without the
precision grip, the delicacy found in the works we see in Lascaux
and Altimira, or for that matter in the works of Poussin, Vermeer,
and Rothko, would never have been possible.

For Fuller, what makes a work of art is that it should imply a
complete symbolic world which can exist independently of the organism's own body but which belongs neither to the organism itself
nor to external reality. Works of art exist, we are reminded, in that
third area of experiencing, neither quite objective nor subjective:
in effect, in potential space where the infant once wilfully imagined
a reality.

By making connections between prehistory and Winnicott's theory of culture and creative living, Fuller argues that he has
constructed a new hypothesis regarding the origins of artistic creativity rooted in materialist knowledge.

THE RENAISSANCE AS A SYMPTOM OF THE REJECTION OF POTENTIAL SPACE

In his *Aesthetics After Modernism*, published the same year as *The Naked Artist*, Fuller applies his hypothesis to the history of art. We thus find:

> If it were permissible to psychologize historical processes, I would say that, in the Renaissance, the 'structure of feeling' changed: emphasis shifted from a sense of fusion with the world (originally the mother) towards 'realistic' individuation, and the recognition of separateness.
>
> (Fuller 1983b: 19)

In the visual arts this shift of emphasis was reflected in the decline of the ornamental and decorative arts and the flowering of the mimetic and figurative arts, because:

> Indeed, one might say that rhythm, pattern and the decorative arts draw upon feelings of union and fusion; whereas carving, figurative painting, and the proportional arts of architecture are rather expressive of separation, and the recognition of the 'other' as an objectively perceived feature.
>
> (Fuller 1983b: 17)

Science was at the root of this shift of emphasis because it led to, amongst other things, the discovery that the world was not created by a feeling mind well-disposed to ourselves, but rather by the chance product of natural processes. From then on, society shifted uneasily between an emotional participation in the world, and the pose that it was outside a system which could be objectively observed.

With the proliferation of industrial capitalism, and the emergence of the 'working class', these developments expunged the 'aesthetic dimension' from everyday life. The division of labour severed the creative relationship between imagination, intellect, heart and hand, so that our 'potential space' began to shrink, and consequently: 'The insult of the Reality Principle impinged deeper and deeper into the lives of ordinary people. There was no room for an intermediate area on production lines, at the pithead, or in steel furnaces' (1983b: 19).

Art persisted nonetheless, but it was no longer an element in our lived relationship to the world; instead it became the pursuit of certain 'creative men of genius' who were set apart in the sense that they were not expected to bow to the inexorable dictates of an increasingly tyrannous Reality Principle. The arts thus became the special preserve for a dimension of imaginative creativity, which had once pervaded all cultural activities, and came to symbolize the celebration of the *illusion* of other realities within the existing one.

Thus, having forsaken decorating architectural space or functional objects, and with the assistance of perspective, the artist became the creator of an illusory space behind the picture frame. In this way, aesthetic form acquired its autonomy from and in fact opposition to, life as lived. In its illusory incarnation behind the picture plane, the 'aesthetic dimension', originally rooted in potential space, disintegrated further by attempting to redeem itself through the Reality Principle – for example, with the advent of naturalism and impressionism. By Late Modernism, defined as 'mainstream' post Second World War art, art had severed itself completely from the 'cosmos of hope' because it ceased to offer 'another reality within the existing one' or a 'miniature realization of the potential space'. The decline continued with functionalist architecture where decoration was outlawed, considered regressive, and so forth.

With Modernist painting, however, we find a temporary reprieve for art because certain painters began to renounce their capacity to create illusory worlds through perspective and the imitation of nature:

> Thus within Modernism, perspective space and the imitation
> of nature fade, and there is a surge of emphasis on painting's
> roots in decoration and sensuous manipulation of materials,
> and a belief that such elements could provide a replacement
> for the lost symbolic order, destroyed by the decline of relig-
> ious iconography, and the subsequent 'failure of nature' to
> provide a substitute.

> (Fuller 1983b: 27)

This mini-revival reached its zenith in Rothko's work, after which most abstract art declined by either pursuing sensuous effects for their own sake, or relinquishing art in favour of the real which, Fuller reminds us, Winnicott considered the 'arch enemy' of creativity (cf. Stephan 1988). By 1969, art was no longer a 'transitional object', a mediator between the real and the 'cosmos of hope', but a mere *thing* indistinguishable from other phenomena. The 'moment of illusion' which good art provides was utterly extinguished; potential space was sealed over even within the practice of painting itself.

THE NECESSITY OF ACCEPTING THE REALITY PRINCIPLE

By asking that we accept his general reference to creativity, thereby not allowing the word to get lost in successful and acclaimed creation, Winnicott clearly acknowledges that his theory makes no claims to explain the possible differences between the construction of art and artefact – the painting as distinct from the hairstyle, for example. Even less so, therefore, can it make claims to explain the creative or aesthetic differences in art practice – music as distinct from literature, painting as distinct from sculpture, for example – or to distinguish between realms – figurative and abstract art, for example.

To my mind, this inability to differentiate suggests a flaw in Winnicott's theory, with its emphasis on creativity. Although it may be that successful infant-mother separation contributes to the constitution of a mentally *healthy* individual and society, it is questionable whether good mothering is a key concept when it comes to accounting for a *creative* individual or society. In fact, the moment Winnicott's admittedly general theory of culture and creative living is applied to specific individuals complications inevitably arise.

For instance, even confining his theory to the fine arts, it is reasonable to assume that those painters who produce prodigious amounts of work contain within themselves a relative excess of creative energy and this is in some way symptomatic of a successful infant-mother relationship. Thus, to take one of many possible examples, Picasso's mother's level of adaption to her infant must have been such that she provided a uniquely fertile area of play. But it can also be argued that Van Gogh's mother's level of adaption must have been equally extraordinary given that her son, at a particular period in his life, also produced a prodigious amount of highly creative work.

Yet according to all accounts, Van Gogh was classifiably mentally ill. Now if Winnicott is right, his illness must have been at least partially contingent upon insensitive mother management, which, in turn, should have afforded him little opportunity for creative development except in terms of introversion or extroversion. It is certainly true that events in Van Gogh's life indicate that there was something of both the introvert and extrovert about the man. He was nonetheless a phenomenally creative individual who, in spite of – or perhaps because of – his mental condition, produced lasting works of creative and currently highly esteemed art.

The point I am making here is that, if both sensitive and insensitive mother management can produce creative beings of the first order, the relevance of the quality of mother management in the first year of a (potential) artist's life as the criterion for the satisfactory development of creativity is severely called into question.

We might, of course, enter into a polemic regarding the respective merits of the art works produced by Picasso and Van Gogh, and perhaps even propose that, whereas Picasso's works are 'healthy' manifestations, those of Van Gogh are not. But even if we adopted this line of questioning, the difficulties in establishing the psychoanalytic criterion for creativity would still remain. That is, is 'unhealthy' art symptomatic of an extraordinary *in*capacity to accept the Reality Principle – a super-charged expression which over-compensates for the strain of relating inner to outer reality? On this assumption, many artists could be accused of failing to accept, more than most, the Reality Principle. But if this were the case then does it necessarily follow that 'healthy' art is a symptom of an *average* incapacity to accept the Reality Principle?

Whatever our personal conclusions may be in this regard, we have seen that Winnicott expressly avoided applying his theory in this way, that is, to make qualitative judgements regarding specific creative realms or realms within realms. (We might, of course, argue that both Picasso's and Van Gogh's exceptional creativity was genetically determined, as was Van Gogh's particular form of insanity – but the emphasis in Winnicott's theory is not on inherited tendencies.)

If Winnicott's theory cannot account for why certain individuals seem to possess a creative excess manifested only in specific realms, even less so can it account for their choice of subject in psychoanalytic terms. For example, are we to believe that Boucher's obvious delight in depicting the sensuous or Goya's capacity to imaginatively and powerfully depict the horrors of war, can be accounted for in terms of a need to produce an adult version of the 'transitional object' symptomatic of a refusal to accept the tyrannous Reality Principle? Surely not, because this type of picture so readily embraces reality. Fuller might not disagree with this but would probably argue that both Boucher and Goya, as post-Renaissance figurative artists, were at fault by creating the illusion of other realities within the existing one.

Before turning to Fuller's hypothesis, further interrelated points can be raised relevant to the underlying premise on which Winnicott bases his theory of culture and creative living. First, why should the average, more or less healthy individual who, through innately determined maturational processes has reached adulthood, not fully come to accept the existence of a separate reality? After all, the whole point of the infant becoming sufficiently cognizant to be able to gain from the experience of frustration is surely precisely to make objects real, thereby affording an understanding enabling successful independent survival throughout life.

Further, while successful infant-mother separation is doubtless important to our development, it has to be contextualized in the light of other important transitional stages in our growth pattern. For example, the advent of puberty often signals the need to seek independence from parental control. This independence typically results in the individual seeking a sexual partner, perhaps eventually marriage and children of his or her own. It is perhaps true to say, by emphasizing that the playing which proceeds from a participation in potential space is genuinely explorative and belongs to health, Winnicott implies that such later transitional processes are normal. Nonetheless, we cannot escape the implication that, because play and the transitional object represent in the infant's mind the *re*union of infant and mother, it is an essentially regressive phenomenon. That is, separation is never fully accepted because no human being is ever free from relating inner to outer reality – with the implication that whatever subsequent developmental stages we experience as a part of our development, these are necessarily coloured by earlier stages and in particular our inability to successfully fully separate from the mother.

In contradiction to Winnicott's views, however, it could be argued that although it is true that 'outer reality' is certainly capable of imposing its fair share of strain, the cause of this imposition typically has a practical basis. Outer reality does not therefore necessarily need to be qualified by contrasting it to an inner reality originally based upon infant-mother fusion and a feeling of omnipotence.

At its most phenomenal, for example, if suddenly caught in a thunderstorm I do not (omnipotently) will the downpour to stop but attempt to shelter to protect myself. If I find no shelter and get soaked I may temporarily object to the Reality Principle but I nonetheless necessarily accept its existence. An infant soaked in a pram may not, of course, and seek protection and compensation in the mother. But this is surely the central difference between infantile and adult responses to the real world.

A second and perhaps more significant point concerns the question: how certain can we be that, in its first year of life, the infant is sufficiently cognizant to be later capable of undergoing potential traumas at the disillusionment stage on becoming aware of a separate reality? This, bearing in mind that at this stage in its development the infant's corpus callosum, along with much else in its brain, is only at incipient stages of its complete maturation. In effect, to what extent is the description disillusionment a tendentious one? After all, it contradictorily implies that, prior to this phase, the infant is to some degree cognizant of the nature of its hallucinating. That is, in order to be *dis*illusioned about something, it is surely necessary to first possess a belief – even if it turns out to be an illusion. And yet the very reason the infant initially experiences 'moments of illusion' is because it is insufficiently mentally developed and therefore incapable of differentiating 'inner' from 'outer' reality.

A CRITIQUE OF PETER FULLER'S ADAPTION OF DONALD WINNICOTT'S THEORY OF CULTURE AND CREATIVE LIVING

If Winnicott expressed reservations about applying his theory of culture and creative living to specific realms of art practice, no such reservations are found in Peter Fuller. I should begin by saying that there is much about Fuller's views I agree with, particularly his emphasis on the effect we, as biological organisms, have in our relations to visual art. I am considerably less certain, however, regarding his free adaption and application of Winnicott's theory to make qualitative judgements in relation to the history of art.

As we saw, Winnicott emphasizes that the creativity which concerns him is universal and it is necessary to separate the idea of creation from the work of art. Fuller, on the other hand, implies that all art practice should be universal in that it should be an element in our lived relations to the world. When art became the pursuit of a few men of genius it inevitably declined. Consequently, whereas one of the difficulties in Winnicott's theory is that it does not attempt to account for works of 'genius', Fuller's solution to the problem is to propose their existence is simply anomalous – in a truly healthy society they would not exist. In this way, it seems to me, he largely avoids having to explain the fact of their existence or their work in psychoanalytic, or, for that matter, any other terms.

Further, the way in which we can distinguish between what might be termed 'integrated' as distinct from 'separatist' art, is by the application of a definite visual criterion underpinned by Winnicott's psychoanalytic theory. For reasons I find unsatisfactory, 'integrated' art is synonymous with decorative and ornamental art because these more readily satisfy the longings we all apparently possess to omnipotently create an imagined reality, thereby refuting the Reality Principle. Figurative and mimetic art, however, while perhaps affording us the illusion of 'other realities within the existing one', is essentially unsatisfactory because its form acquiesces to the tyrannous Reality Principle. This is because, as far as I can make out, figurative art attempts, amongst other things, to accurately copy nature and, with the aid of perspective, to place its subject 'behind' the picture plane. Because of this it forfeits the possibility of existing as an element in our lived relationship with the world but, on the contrary, constitutes an opposition to life as lived.

This has the implication that the closer visual art becomes to representing the world as it is more or less actually perceived because of the biological structure of our visual system, the more it acquiesces to the tyrannous Reality Principle and the less psychologically valid it becomes. This is mainly because the figurative strays from the true purpose of art, namely, providing an intermediate area thereby affording us relief from the strain of relating inner to outer reality. From this it follows that both Boucher's *Reclining Girl* and Goya's *3rd May 1808*, constitute 'bad' art because they are too readily reminiscent of the real, phenomenally imposing world.

The decline of 'good' art, we are informed, began with the Renaissance when, primarily because of science, society became (cognitively) split between an emotional participation in the world and the tendency to delude itself that the world could be objectively viewed. This manifested itself in the decline of the ornamental and decorative arts with their emphasis on rhythm and pattern which are equated with infant-mother fusion, the 'aesthetic dimension', potential space, and the transitional object. These were (unfortunately) ousted by the mimetic arts including carving, figurative painting and the proportional arts of architecture, all symptomatic of infant-mother separation and the recognition of the 'other' as an objectively perceived feature.

However, if the decline of good art began at the Renaissance with its flowering of figurative and mimetic art symptomatic of the rejection of potential space, we should be able to assume with some certainty that, prior to the Renaissance, art exhibited no such characteristics. Also, art produced as a result of and concomitant with the phylogenetic emergence of potential space should *certainly* not exhibit characteristics symptomatic of its rejection. That is, art produced in virtue of the neoteny phenomenon should have been ornamental and decorative with an emphasis on pattern and rhythm, thereby reflecting the importance of the infant-mother relationship (only recently) afforded by attenuated growth.

The evidence dictates, however, that this is simply not the case as Fuller, if paradoxically, is the first to admit. We thus find him proposing that even before the advent of neoteny:

> With Neanderthal man, we find evidence of burial rites, and
> simple carvings incorporating unmistakable bodily and sexual
> symbolism, and even representations of animals in painting
> and engraving which we first came across a little before
> 30,000BC. Then, suddenly, there is an efflorescence of cultu-
> ral activity evidenced in those famous prehistoric cave paint-
> ings which belong to a period between 30,000 and about
> 8,000BC.

(Fuller 1983a: 12)

Two of these paintings have already been referred to in this book – a bison and a reindeer found in the caves of Altamira and Font de Gaume – also, a horse statuette from the Vogelherd dated 29,000 BC. Whatever their original symbolic usage, all of these

198

image forms are clearly figurative and mimetic. This they should not be, according to Fuller's hypothesis, because figurative and mimetic art is symptomatic of our species' (misguided) pose, adopted at the Renaissance, that we are outside a system capable of being objectively observed.

And here we can be reminded that the whole point of Marshack's paper, reviewed in chapter 3.2, was to investigate how the late Neanderthal came to divorce and symbolize the greater, natural environment from the self. In relation to the statuettes found at Vogelherd, for example, Marshack could propose that they indicated a cognitive capacity for abstraction, modelling, and the manufacture of a different order than that which could be deduced from the subsistence tool industries. Part of this different order manifested itself in the protolinguistic marks carved into the figurative statuettes. These marks – which might superficially appear purely decorative and ornamental – in fact, says Marshack, indicate the presence of a tradition of non-representational symbolic markings that may have required some form of linguistic explanation.

In effect, the figurative image, carved from stone or bone and a mimetic reminder of the phenomenal world, provided the Neanderthal with a culturally manufactured context from which to abstract. I could thus propose earlier, 'if the artifacts are seen as a symptom of our emerging capacity to abstract and conceptualize, it must have developed concomitant with our capacity to rationalize both our environment and personal status. This in turn suggests a degree of self-awareness and therefore an emerging capacity to differentiate ourselves as a species' (3.6).

From this it follows that the seeds of our shift from a sense of fusion with the world (originally the mother) towards a 'realistic' individuation and the recognition of our separateness, began not at the Renaissance, as Fuller proposes, but no later than with the Neanderthal.

If we therefore logically pursue Fuller's argument that figurative and mimetic art is 'bad' art because, by accepting the Reality Principle, it loses its power to become an element in our lived relationship with the world, we arrive at the following *non sequitur*. The decline of good art began with its cause, that is, potential space contingent upon attenuated growth afforded by neoteny. Put differently, concomitant with the origins of our tendency to create integrated art because of prolonged infant-mother dependence, we find the production of a class of imagery expressive of separation and the recognition of the 'other' as an objectively perceived feature.

At this point, then, Fuller's psychoanalytically based hypothesis, which is so reliant upon phylogenetically substantiating the role potential space plays in the differentiation of classes of art, is severely challenged. This is partially because the moment we concentrate on the possible *reasons* for neoteny, rather than the phenomenon itself, it becomes no more than a secondary symptom of our cognitive evolution as a species, not a cause.

Fuller thus argues that the most extraordinary fact about late Neanderthals was their large brain size which constituted a predicament for mothers with too small pelvic structures. However, nothing is mentioned from a cognitive perspective about *why* it might have been that brain size suddenly increased, with the exception of the reference:

> Neoteny (combined, no doubt, with the neurological evolution of the brain) enriched humanity's psychological processes, endowed us with the capacity for symbolic and imaginative thought, and gave rise to a dream life fuller than that of any other species.
>
> (Fuller 1983a: 18)

Surely, however, it was the neurological evolution of the brain prior to neoteny which caused it, and it is therefore surely the reason why the brain suddenly 'exploded' prior to neoteny which most deserves our attention. That is, although neoteny doubtlessly played its part in the evolution of our species, its significance lies in its secondary role as an adaptive symptom of an already expanding cognitive capacity. Attempting to understand the nature of this capacity and the part it plays in creativity and the production of different classes of art, by referring to the size of the Neanderthal infant's skull, is a bit like trying to deduce the workings of a car engine by analysing its bonnet.

Fuller's argument is, of course, that neoteny led to attenuated growth and prolonged infant-mother reliance thereby allowing the infant's imagination to acquire an infinitely labile, transforming and world creating quality, etc. However, the way in which this uniquely human capacity developed, is described in the vaguest of Winnicottian terms with the odd reference to Darwin and Marx: 'Darwin and Marx recognized this peculiar quality of the imagin-

ation as *the* decisive human factor ... we have been taking it down
to its biological roots' (1983a: 17).

No effort is made to investigate in depth the class of symbol form
through which imagination manifests itself, and consequently no
conclusions can be drawn regarding the nature of the respective
communicative potentials associated with different symbol systems,
the part they play in child development, the differences between
the production and perception of art, and so forth.

An example of this failure to differentiate is reflected in Fuller's
proposal that the illusion provided by perspective at the Renaissance was a symptom of science which led to art no longer being
an element in our lived relationship to the world. Granted, however, that the production of figurative imagery aided by perspective
has something of the scientific about it, it does not mean that our
response is scientifically governed – any more than it is in relation
to the pictures afforded us by the technological innovation of tele-
vision.

Perhaps the most serious criticism regarding the psychoanalytic
component of Fuller's hypothesis, presents itself in the form of fact,
however. Even the cultural products of the Neanderthal and Cromagnon excepted, it is palpably true that 'illusionism' has been with
us not merely since the Renaissance, but existed at least 1,500 years
earlier in Greek art. Gombrich can thus propose:

> The stylistic changes in Greek art from the archaic repre-
> sentations of the sixth century to the illusionistic illustrations
> of the third constitute the most famous advance of this kind,
> which was recapitulated in the Renaissance development
> from Giotto to Leonardo da Vinci.
>
> (Gombrich 1979: 80)

Gombrich continues by informing us how naturalistic inventions
spread with the same rapidity as other technical innovations, 'The
mastery of the nude in Greek art impressed sculptors as far as Af-
ghanistan and Gandhara; the invention of perspective in Florence
conquered France and Germany within a century' (1979: 80).

In my view, the reason why these 'naturalistic inventions' spread
with such rapidity is because they constitute a visual truth, namely,
they correspond in certain essentials to how our optical system
allows us to visually perceive the world, as I have argued at length.
Surely, then, our acceptance of this truth is more realistic and con-

structive than attempting to criticize it on the grounds of its failure to re-kindle in the adult infantile longings to imagine reality at will; grounds which, as we saw, when traced to their possible phylogeny, become self-contradictory.

But even if it were accepted that neoteny, and therefore in Fuller's terms 'potential space', played their part in prehistoric art, because 'illusionism' has been with us for a minimum of 2,000 years, it must surely be accepted as constituting a valid art form. If this means that for over 2,000 years we have succumbed to the tyrannous Reality Principle and have, therefore, in some way collectively rejected the implications of 'potential space' (albeit before its conceptualization by Winnicott), this is surely symptomatic of the direction of our cognitive and social development as a species. A direction currently expressing itself in the visual arts by, through the use of film and video, a need to embrace more than ever the Reality Principle. Film and video offers us not only 'pictures' but movement and sound; holography promises a lot more.

From this perspective, representational painting's acceptance of the Reality Principle does not mean that it is a failed 'transitional object', but, on the contrary, possibly a forerunner of our species' attempt to construct equivalents for our capacity to intersensorially perceive phenomena. On this premise the representational image clearly fails to properly realize the Reality Principle simply because its version of the phenomenal world is confined to a petrification of only one of its aspects, the visual. This is why I can propose that the representational visual image exists in a (psychological) equivocal reality, that is, one lying between its potential to 'trigger' our biologically/cognitively processed lived experience of reality, and its material incapacity to resolve this reality. In this phenomenally and neuropsychologically underpinned sense, art indeed belongs neither to the organism itself nor to external reality – simply because, as biological organisms, we can only inadequately participate in the reality proposed.

In contrast to Fuller's hypothesis, then, my own begins with the assumption that the percipient of representational imagery comes to it fully accepting the Reality Principle and thereafter responds to its incapacity to resolve the very reality it so readily suggests. In this way, pictures indeed do always exist on the theoretical line between the subjective and the objective – but this position is not traceable to the hypothetical area that exists between the infant and its object (mother or part-mother) during the phase of repudiation of the object as 'not-me'. The ambiguity in pictures is more pragmatically traceable to the phenomenally related discrepancy between what is objectively visually perceived and what is subjectively known about a picture's referents.

This is not to assume that the cognitive rift that may result from the effects of experiencing this phenomenally based discrepancy cannot trigger, in relation to certain pictures and individuals, all manner of psychoanalytically classifiable responses. Nor is it to assume that certain pictures cannot explicitly suggest the infant-mother relationship, as in the case of Madonna pictures.

NOTES

INTRODUCTION

1   Founded in 1966 by Nelson Goodman, who was succeeded by
    Howard Gardner and David Perkins, and then Gardner, Harvard
    Project Zero is a collaboration of individuals concerned with the
    nature of cognition, symbol processing, and their possible
    relations to the arts and education. Cf. Perkins and Leondar,
    1977: 1–4. For Gombrich's views, see Gombrich, 1979: 184–8.
2   I am using 'art theoretician' to denote, in a general sense, those
    who in some way linguistically comment upon the visual arts. I
    am not, therefore, for the present distinguishing between art
    critics, aestheticians, semioticians, or historians, for example.
3   The view that visual art, and in particular the representational
    visual image, is capable of communicating its message without
    linguistic intervention, is by no means given, as we shall see
    presently regarding the views of Barthes and Panofsky in
    particular.
4   For those who follow Chomsky, it could be argued that language
    grammars are a finite means of generating an infinity of
    sentences.
5   For Barthes, the linguistic message functions in terms of *anchorage*
    and *relay*, devices which guide our understanding of the visual
    image, which is *polysemous*, i.e. underlying the signifiers of all
    visual images is a 'floating chain' of signifieds or different
    meanings. Linguistic description therefore 'anchors' the meaning
    of an image, thereby directing us to a 'correct' level of perception
    and understanding. Cf. Barthes 1982: 38–41.
6   Gardner proposes that the attempt to understand rapidly processed
    and sometimes 'nonconscious' information is current among
    information-processing psychology or cognitive science research,
    and therefore:

> A researcher working in the information processing paradigm
> seeks to provide a second-by-second (or even a millisecond-by-
> millisecond) 'microgenetic' picture of the mental steps involved

as a child solves (or fails to solve) a conservation problem....
Such a descriptive *tour de force* involves detailed analysis of the
task itself, as well as painstaking analysis of the subject's
thoughts and behaviour.

(Gardner 1984: 22)

7   Although the corpus callosum is the hemispheres' major
communication pathway, other lesser pathways also exist. The
functional role of the corpus callosum is described in my opening
chapter.

8   Regarding research concentrating on left-hemisphere function,
Gardner *et al.* comment:

Language has almost universally been considered the most
central human cognitive capacity; and, more so than any other
function, language seems (in normal right-handers) to be lateralized to the left cerebral cortex... Thus, although hardly ever
tested in a thorough manner, the idea persisted that an individual's cognitive competence is closely linked to the inactness of
his left hemisphere, as did the corollary assumption that individuals with right-hemisphere damage, their language apparently
intact, are not seriously compromised in their ability to understand situations, solve problems, and make their way in the
world.

(Gardner *et al.* 1983: 171)

9   Gazzaniga is clearly indicating a modular view of mental activity,
currently undergoing a revival in faculty psychology. The
subsumption of nonverbal ways of knowing by linguistic ones has
led certain researchers to conclude that hemispheric specialization
challenges the unity of consciousness by suggesting the existence
of at least two centres of consciousness existing in a single body.
Others, less extreme, argue that the idea of mental unity is not
seriously challenged because, with the exception of the brain-
damaged, the hemispheres are functionally integrated. For a
review of some of the arguments, see Nagel (1971) and Sperry
(1983).
    My own view is that the results of lateralization research
clearly indicate a degree of modularity which could easily go
unacknowledged because we speak in the first person singular and
therefore tend to assume that our mental unity is in some way
absolute.

10   Warrington and Taylor (1973, 1978) have published findings which
indicate that the right parietal lobe is crucial in the recognition of
objects perceived from unconventional views, as we shall see in
chapter 3.3.

11   My theory, which takes into account our evolution, experience and
cognition, shares aspects in common with Berleant's (1970)
phenomenological approach to aesthetics which argues that art

has deep biological roots, that aesthetic theory should be developed as a cognitive discipline, that aspects of art are materially explicable, and so forth.

12   I return to the reasons for the representational image's ability to sustain its full existential life (in spite of our better knowledge), thereby potentially generating certain response tendencies, in chapters 3, 4, and 7 in particular.

1   THE BIOLOGICAL AND PROCEDURAL BASES OF NEUROPSYCHOLOGY

1   The left and right cerebral hemispheres of the brain are connected by the corpus callosum, a large band of nerve fibres which allow higher order information to be exchanged in some form between the hemispheres. In split-brain surgery the corpus callosum is often completely sectioned, typically as a last resort for intractable epilepsy. The majority of the split-brain or commissurotomy operations occurred in the 1960s. Since then several neuro-surgeons have attempted to control intractable epilepsy by limiting surgery to those areas of the corpus callosum and anterior commissures most likely to transmit epileptic discharges. (Cf. Risse *et al.* 1977; LeDoux *et al.* 1977a, 1977b)

2   Gazzaniga (1970) describes how one of his commissurotomy sub-jects, when attempting to put on his trousers, found his left hand struggling against the right. One hand attempted to pull them up while the other pull them down. In another incident, when the subject became angry, he aggressively reached for his wife with his left hand which was subsequently held by the right in an attempt to control it.

3   Personal correspondence with Michael Youngblood is found in chapter 6, note 14.

4   Each lobe is known to serve a different sensory or motor function. The occipital lobe is a visual centre whereas parts of the temporal lobe are involved in audition. The anterior part of the parietal lobe is concerned with somatosensory function, and parts of the lobe are concerned with spatial processing. The posterior part of the frontal lobe mediates certain motor functions. The areas of the cortex which receive inputs from the sense organs or which control movements of particular parts of the body, are known as primary zones or primary projection areas. The primary areas in the parietal, temporal, and occipital lobes are known to possess high modal or domain specificity. In higher animals, and par-ticularly our species, however, much of the cortex is not obviously committed to specific senses and these areas are consequently known as 'secondary association' areas. For a detailed description of the lobes and their possible functions, see Dimond (1978: 57–73).

5   The isolation of the hemispheres is not absolute because various unifying functions are retained which appear to compensate for the absence of the corpus callosum. Conjugate eye movements and the fact that information from each eye is registered by both hemispheres, establishes a degree of unity in the visual realm. The ipsilateral and contralateral pathways from the ears establish a unit in the auditory realm. There is also evidence to suggest that (weaker) ipsilateral as well as contralateral pathways exist in the touch modality. It has also been suggested that some information, particularly of an emotional origin, may be made available to both hemispheres via the lower brain stem commissures which lie well below the cortex. (Cf. Sperry *et al.* 1979). Regarding emotion in particular, see Mandler (1975) and note 7 of this chapter.

6   The visual pathways to the respective hemispheres are not interfered with in the commissurotomy operation.

7   A possible origin of the current use of 'cross-modal' comes from the research of Norman Geschwind. In a recent review of his work, Rosenfield points out:

> Instead of the direct connections between auditory or visual information and limbic responses that are characteristic of animals, human beings have powerful associations between visual and auditory sensations as well as between the tactile and the auditory, the tactile and the visual, etc... Geschwind called them 'cross-modal' associations. As he wrote: 'In sub-human forms the only readily established sensory–sensory associations are those between non-limbic (i.e. visual, tactile or auditory) stimulus and a limbic (fight, flight or sexual) response. It is only in man that associations between two non-limbic stimuli are readily formed'.
>
> (Rosenfield 1985: 50–1)

The limbic system, which exists in the midbrain and is covered by the cortex, and whose evolutionary development pre-dates the cortex, is associated with the control of instinctive and emotional behaviour. The hypothalamus, which constitutes a part of the limbic system, is concerned with the regulation of the autonomic nervous system.

8   Although there is evidence to suggest that (weaker) ipsilateral pathways exist in the touch modality, these appear to be relatively insensitive. Researchers therefore asked subjects to use their left hand because of its stronger contralateral neural connections to the right (nonverbal) hemisphere, which, it was assumed, had exclusively received the tachistoscopically presented information and would, therefore, be capable of a response.

9   If we include the commissurotomized as 'brain-damaged', then the same rule applies to their auditory system as it did to the visual system, i.e. the auditory pathways to the hemispheres are not interfered with in the commissurotomy operation (see note 6.) If,

however, the subject has suffered damage to the left temporal lobe, for example, it may be the case that the damage inhibits the registration and processing of a given auditory stimulus (see note 4).

10 The fact that spoken *digits* were used could appear confusing in that they introduce a mathematical as distinct from a linguistic dimension to the test. The test was, however, designed to illuminate the hemispheres' linguistic, not their mathematical potential.

11 Galin and Ornstein's proposal that in the majority of ordinary activities we alternate between the cognitive modes associated with the respective hemispheres, complements Jerre Levy's (1969) conclusions regarding the evolution of cerebral asymmetry of function. She argues that the respective hemispheres evolved distinct modes of cognitive processing to minimize mutual interference. Levy's views complement those of Marr concerning his 'principle of modular design', as well as my own, as we shall see in chapter 3.

12 Brain rhythms have been described as falling into four distinct categories: beta, alpha, theta and delta. Beta rhythms are associated with concentrated brain activity, alpha rhythms with relaxed mental states, and theta and delta with sleep states.

2 THE EXPERIMENTAL EVIDENCE

1 Gazzaniga and LeDoux note that while the term 'manipulospatial' is used to describe activities that would otherwise be called motor and perceptual functions, they feel that the idea of a manipulospatial mechanism transcends these simple notions. They view manipulospatial function as the mechanism by which a spatial context is mapped onto the perceptual and motor activities of the hands. On the efferent side, the activities involved in drawing, arranging, constructing, or otherwise manipulating items; on the afferent side, the active, exploratory manipulations involved in the evaluation of the spatiotemporal features of complex haptic stimuli. (Cf. Gazzaniga and LeDoux 1978: 55–6)

2 Before Broca's seminal paper (1861), Marc Dax hypothesized that speech was confined to the left hemisphere. His hypothesis resulted from observations of over forty patients suffering from aphasia. He could not, however, provide clinical data to support his hypothesis. It can also be noted that Franz Gall proposed that the brain is not a uniform mass and that mental faculties can be cerebrally localized. He too could not provide clinical data to substantiate his claims.

3 Research that concentrated on aphasic disabilities, primarily associated with the left hemisphere, often illuminated by second intention the possible nature of right-hemisphere function. (Cf.

Brain 1941; Battersby *et al.* 1956)

4   Sperry's argument is that because the left hemisphere was not cognizant of higher level mental performances exhibited by the right hemisphere in the experimental situation, it is unlikely to have contributed to their realization. The implication is that the right hemisphere is capable of a high level of independent performance.

5   I deal more comprehensively with the question of right-hemisphere consciousness in chapter 4, by which time most of the relevant data will have been reviewed. It is nonetheless worth noting that by the late 1960s there were clear signs that Sperry and Gazzaniga were beginning to regard the conscious status of the right hemisphere in a different light. This should become more obvious later in this chapter when I review two seminal experiments respectively conducted by Sperry and Gazzaniga.

6   Some of the research was conducted with Sperry.

7   Gazzaniga and LeDoux propose that, rather than drawing tests pointing to a right-hemisphere advantage *per se* relative to the left in spatial programming, it could be that the left has difficulty in representing 'spatiality' using a manual or manipulative response.

8   The subjects were classified as follows:

    293   right-handers with left-brain lesions
    194   right-handers with right-brain lesions
     47   left-handers with left brain lesions
     26   left-handers with right-brain lesions

9   The fact that subjects used both left and right hands to point to right-hemisphere registered stimuli provides evidence that the right hemisphere can control the right as well as the left hand in simple pointing tasks. The implication is that some ipsilateral fibres exist to allow each hemisphere to exert some control on the same side of the body. It is generally acknowledged, however, that ipsilateral motor control is generally coarse and limited to movements of the whole of the arm or hand. (See chapter 1.2)

10   The assumption here is that the respective halves of any one face in some way visually express the workings of the contralateral hemisphere. It should be noted, however, that the musculature necessary for facial expression is to some degree controlled by both hemispheres. (See chapter 1.2)

11   The researchers' belief that P.S. was the *first* split-brain subject to possess double consciousness clearly contradicts the conclusion reached by Sperry eleven years previously, i.e. that in the split-brain we deal with two separate spheres of consciousness, etc. (Cf. Sperry 1968)

12   Regarding the nature of the mental aura, Sperry *et al.* later note:

    Questions remain also about the nature, mechanisms and functional role of the emotional and mental aura generated by the perception and recognition of a key test item. At least large components of the aura seemed to spread readily to the opposite hemisphere presumably through the brain stem systems. In addition to general emotional changes the central transfer appeared to include also subtle cognitive effects that enabled categorical distinctions like those between government and personal, domestic vs foreign, historical vs entertainment, etc. Common experience suggests that such emotional and conative auras play an important orientational role in normal brain function, as, for example, mnemonic retrieval.

(Sperry *et al.* 1979: 165)

It is also worth noting that in tests conducted on the subject P.S., Gazzaniga and LeDoux record that unilaterally right-hemisphere registered information of an emotional and conative class appeared to 'leak', in a directionally specific manner, to the left hemisphere. The left hemisphere could not, however, verbally identify the nature of the information. For example, on a verbal command test, the word *kiss* was lateralized to P.S.'s right hemisphere, immediately after which his left hemisphere blurted out, 'Hey, no way, no way, no way. You've got to be kidding.' When asked what it was he was not going to do, P.S. was unable to tell the examiners. (Cf. Gazzaniga and LeDoux 1978: 151–5) I return to the significance of these tests on the arts and cognition in chapters 4.4, 4.5, 7.7, and 7.8.

13 Bever explains the right-ear effect as follows: 'Our interpretation has been that musicians have learned to listen to music in an analytic way which stimulates the kind of processing natural to the left hemisphere' (Bever 1983: 23). Bever's proposal makes good sense because a professional musician necessarily *reads* a musical score in something like the way in which we read language (sequentially, from left to right, etc.).

3 THE POSSIBLE ORIGINS OF CEREBRAL SPECIALIZATION

1 As to exactly why prehistorical humans used the right hand in the first place is not known. It is worth noting, however, that Needham (1982) proposes that the neonate naturally sought the pulse of the maternal heart. From this it is concluded that in prehistory both maternal nurturing and infantile orienting reactions tended to behaviourally reinforce the efficiency of sequential operations in the left hemisphere.

2 The term 'hardwired' comes from current computer science and artificial intelligence research and describes the neurons or electric circuits in the brain which allow mental procedures to be effected.

3   This view that language developed as a consequence of different
     sensory associations parallels Gazzaniga's (ontogenetic) view that
     when the child explores with the right hand, visual, auditory, or
     tactile engrams become established in the left hemisphere,
     reviewed in section 4 of this chapter. Also see chapter 1, notes 4
     and 7.

4   Both Marshack and Marr are adopting a perspective known to
     philosophers as *evolutionary epistemology*. (Cf. Hookway 1984)

5   As early as 1959, Lettvin published a classic paper which argued
     that the frog's eye tells it four things. Whether there are any
     sustained contrasts, convexities, dark edges and whether there is a
     net darkening over the bulk of the field. From this Lettvin
     concluded that the eye speaks to the brain in a language already
     highly organized and interpreted, instead of transmitting some
     more or less accurate copy of what is seen. In the same year as
     Lettvin's paper, Hubel and Wiesel (1959) published evidence to
     suggest that the visual cortex of the cat also extracts features from
     the environment, notably straight lines of definite length and
     orientation. Finally, it is worth noting that earlier research by
     Hartline and Barlow had predicted the above contributions to
     vision by showing that the eye of the horseshoe crab has on/off
     detectors (Hartline 1942).

6   Strictly speaking, then, Marr's theory does not apply to asym-
     metrical objects.

7   This conclusion is important to theories of picture perception
     because it implies that we do not need to *learn* to see pictures and
     therefore argues against the view that pictures are mere
     conventions. I return to theories of picture perception in chapter
     6.

8   This process is sometimes referred to as *neoteny*, the process by
     which one or more of the early stages and features in the
     development of an animal are retained into later periods of
     growth.

9   Regarding the mutually reinforcing right-hand/left-hemisphere
     relationship, Kimura and Archibald (1974) have proposed that
     left-hemisphere specialization for speech is a consequence of
     certain motor skills that happen to lend themselves to
     communication. From this it follows that the left hemisphere
     evolved language, not because it became more 'symbolic' or
     analytic, but because it became well adapted to certain categories
     of motor activity.

10   This view is supported by Warrington and Taylor when, concerning
     right- and left-hemisphere damaged subjects' capacities to
     recognize objects, they propose:

         The right-hemisphere group was significantly worse than the
         left-hemisphere group in recognizing the unconventional view
         objects, and the right posterior group obtained the highest

error score and was significantly worse than the left posterior group. Yet in the conventional view there was no impairment in any patient group.

(Warrington and Taylor 1973: 162)

As implied by the above, the researchers succeeded in locating the capacity to recognize 'unconventional view' objects not only to the right hemisphere, but to its parietal lobe.

11   Regarding the quasi-iconic nature of certain pictorial stimuli forms, see the distinctions Pateman (1986) draws between transparent and translucent icons.

4   THE RIGHT-HEMISPHERE COGNITIVE PARADIGM

1   Although the capacity to causally link paralinguistic sound phenomena to a concrete referent is an intuitive (unlearned) process, the capacity to *name* the phenomena in the relation (*barking/dog*) clearly is a learned process.

2   We do not need to be skilled in drawing techniques to take photographs which incorporate sophisticated rules of perspective.

3   As we shall see presently regarding Panofsky's views, it is by no means given that we are capable of properly appreciating certain art works without some prior learned and linguistically imparted knowledge.

4   I have borrowed the term intersensorial from Piaget (1966: 75, for example).

5   It is still open to question how choices of this kind, which work at speed and appear to involve complex cognitive processes, are made. Computer scientists often embrace the assumption that we run at incredible speed through a series of calculations that would demand an enormous amount of programming for a computer to perform a similar task. Dreyfus (1972), on the other hand, proposes that it is our status as sensory beings which enables us to perform apparently complex calculations at speed, as we shall see later in this chapter.

6   One of the reasons, in my view, that Fodor's account of our mental structures is convincing is because it closely resembles Geschwind's neurological account of how we deal with information. Geschwind concluded that in both higher animals and human beings, sensory information (from Fodor's *transducers*) is initially processed in the primary sensory areas of the brain. The information is then related to neighbouring brain regions known as association areas. In higher animals, but not in humans, the information then passes to the limbic system, an area that activates emotional responses such as fight, flight, and sexual approach. In human beings, information from the association areas can bypass the limbic system to be processed by the

secondary association areas (Fodor's *central systems*). These secondary association areas free our species from domination by the limbic system responses, thereby, in one sense, allowing us to 'think' before we may act. (Cf. Geschwind 1974: 105–236)

7 Pucetti (1973, 1976) and Bogen (1969b) have inferred from the clinical data that each hemisphere has a 'mind' of its own – not only after brain bisection but also in the normal (intact) state. The logic of such arguments typically goes as follows. If cutting the cross-connections between the hemispheres leaves two co-conscious mental systems, then there must have existed two independently operating systems to begin with.

8 It can be hypothesized further that the right hemisphere had three units of information from which to construct a best available hypothesis as to why the chicken head was chosen, i.e. a snow scene, shovel and chicken head. If it so happened that the right hemisphere did construct a hypothesis, it can be assumed that it could not be (verbally) communicated because of its lack of speech centres.

9 Research by Kennedy (1974, 1977) on the blind indicates that their sense of touch allows them a remarkably well-developed sense of the nature of spatial relations. Also see Pateman (1986).

10 Gazzaniga currently views much of split-brain research as a technique to expose modularity. We thus find:

> We begin to see that the brain has a modular nature, a point that comes out of all the data. It is of only secondary interest that the modules should always be in the same place. A correlate of this is that much of split-brain research should be viewed as a technique to expose modularity. That is, it is not important that the left brain does this or the right brain does that. But it is highly interesting that by studying patients with their cerebral hemispheres separated certain mental skills can be observed in isolation.
>
> (Gazzaniga 1985: 58–9)

11 Also see Introduction to this book, notes 8 and 9.
12 I develop the implications of the view that pictures exist in their own space and time continuum in chapter 7.

5 CHILDREN'S DRAWING

1 By emphasizing this reciprocity Piaget distinguishes himself from the associationists who propose that stimulus response is a one-way process, and also from those who Piaget calls 'theorists of form' (Chomsky and Fodor, for example) who, essentially disregarding the part experience plays in our development, believe that internal maturation of cognitive structures is alone capable of explaining their progressive coherence. Nonetheless,

Selfe argues that Piaget pays insufficient attention to the influence experience plays in the development of the child because he:

> talks as if the child creates the real world without either an interaction between the child and his environment or even that environment impinging on the child to alter the course of his development.... His system is metaphysical rather than scientific and Piaget constructs a model in which the pinnacle of development is logical deductive thinking.
>
> (Selfe 1985: 16)

2   Compare with chapter 3.2 regarding our phylogeny and capacity to symbol form.
3   Given the difficulties surrounding the mental image because of its internalization, Piaget has no empirical means of substantiating that it becomes active only at the semiotic period. For more recent accounts of the mental image, see Block (1981) and Selfe (1983).
4   It is perhaps tendentious to propose that one stage is a failed version of another. Arnheim (1974), for example, argues that it is a mistake to call a child's drawing distorted or deformed because it does not accord with visual reality.
5   But see what Boden (1979) says about Piaget's 'Achilles Heel' when she analyses the way in which paraplegics cope with the world.
6   I substantiate the view that there is such a thing as an 'objective' visual reality in chapter 6 when examining theories of picture perception.
7   Korzenik proposes that decontextualization requires the ability to look at one's behaviour as others may see it; to be able to conceive of a viewpoint different to one's own.
8   Arnheim (1974) would argue that this is a perfectly reasonable interpretation of a child's visual experience of a house because things are rarely viewed statically. Therefore, since many views of an object are possible then many spatial relationships can be represented in a drawing.

In my view, Arnheim is mistaken, however, because whereas in real life we may be confronted with constantly changing views of an object, such is the nature of our visual system that we cannot see them all at once. That is, any object or scene is always viewed from a fixed perspective at any one moment in virtue of our bodily position in space and time. As we walk down a road the view will, of course, change – the view perceived half-way down will not be the same as the one perceived at its beginning. If, however, half-way down the view perceived at its beginning were registered along with the present view, we would become disoriented. The same is generally true when our visual system is presented with a multi-dimensional view of an object or scene represented in two dimensions.

Arnheim is therefore confusing the multi-dimensional views often presented in children's drawing as being a true *visual* experience of an object or scene (which it is not), with it being a legitimate *conceptual* representation of an object or scene (which it can be).

9 By 'communicative' part of the human anatomy I simply mean that, in addition to it being able to communicate a subtle range of expressions and emotions, the head is the only part that contains all five senses.

10 Here it is worth again referring to Marr's views reviewed in chapter 3.3 that parts of the visual image that we can name and which have a meaning for us, do not necessarily have distinctive characteristics that can be uniquely specified in a computer program. Thus, the same circle could represent a wheel, the sun, or a table-top contingent upon the context of the situation. I have recalled these views because it seems to me that the reason a computer program is incapable of correctly contextualizing certain shapes – whereas children are – is simply because it lacks the capacity to experientially understand what a shape's referent might be *vis-à-vis* other shapes in the world. Put differently, it cannot contextualize certain shapes by referring them to their broader, life-associated context.

11 Aspects of the mental strategy employed by children at the *failed realism* stage could share something in common with those employed by the right-hemisphere damaged subjects referred to in chapter 3.6; that is, their drawing revealed an almost exclusive dependence on a propositional knowledge of the subject, its name and features.

6 THE LANGUAGES OF ART

1 This does not mean that conventional theories necessarily insist that we need to learn to see pictures in the same way that we learn to read a language; rather, the connection is typically only implied.

> The temptation is to call a system of depiction a language; but here I stop short. The question what distinguishes representational from linguistic systems needs close examination. One might suppose that the criterion of realism can be made to serve here too; that symbols grade from the most realistic depictions through less and less realistic ones to descriptions. This is surely not the case; the measure of realism is habituation, but descriptions do not become depictions by habituation. The most commonplace nouns of English have not become pictures.
>
> (Goodman 1968: 41)

Goodman argues elsewhere:

> Nothing is intrinsically a representation; status as representation is relative to symbol system. A picture in one system

may be a description in another; and whether a denoting system is representational depends not upon whether it resembles
what it denotes but upon its own relationships to other symbols
in a given scheme.

(Goodman 1968: 226)

2   In contradiction to this view, as early as 1937 Nadel showed that
     people from widely different cultures recognize pictures in
     common ways. Thus both the Yoruba and Nubes people of
     Nigeria experienced little difficulty in identifying photographs of
     men, animals and a bush fire. This was in spite of the fact that the
     Yoruba's art consisted mainly of wooden images and hand-made
     pictures, whereas the Nube's art consisted of decorative and
     ornamental forms. (Cf. Nadel 1937)
3   Gombrich's views on picture perception are at times ambiguous.
     Thus, whereas in the view just quoted he implies that our ability
     to relate to pictures is an innately determined capacity, elsewhere
     he emphasizes the conventional theory (1977: 55–7, for example).
     In fact, Eco refers to this particular section of Gombrich's book to
     substantiate his own conventionalist argument (Eco 1979: 204–5).
     For further views on Gombrich's position, see Hogg (1969).
4   In a study by Hohmann (1966) the question was asked whether
     visceral response is necessary for emotional experience. Subjects
     with varying degrees of spinal cord injuries were divided into five
     groups according to the degree of visceral innervation on the
     assumption that the higher the spinal cord injury, the less
     powerful emotional sensations would be (simply because of the
     increasing lack of connection between brain and body).
        Various forms of stimuli, including visual erotica, were
     presented to the subjects with the purpose of provoking states of
     excitement. It was concluded that the higher the spinal cord injury
     the greater was the loss of response. I have referred to this study
     because it indicates that our response to at least certain forms of
     pictorial stimuli is inextricably linked to our biology.
5   Here, it is worth noting Panofsky's views on the ways in which
     various cultures emphasize different aspects of form:

When we call a figure in an Italian Renaissance picture 'plastic'
while describing a picture in a Chinese painting as 'having vol-
ume but no mass' (owing to the absence of modelling), we
interpret these figures as two different solutions of a problem
which might be formulated as 'volumetric units (bodies) *vs.* il-
limited expanse (space).' ... Upon reflection it will turn out that
there is a limited number of such primary problems, interrelated with each other, which on the one hand beget an
infinity of secondary and tertiary ones, and on the other hand
can be ultimately derived from one basic antithesis: differentiation *vs.* continuity.

(Panofsky 1955: 21)

6　In this instance, Panofsky's view can be compared to those of Barthes as found in note 5 of my introduction to this book.

7　It can be noted here that I am developing a 'sensuous-naturalist' view of art as distinct from a 'conceptualist-idealist' one.

8　It should be emphasized that I am not arguing that art history has no validity as a discipline in its own right as a specialized branch of history. My objection concerns the insistence that a sophisticated knowledge of art history is necessary to 'correct' a perhaps more intuitive response to pictures.

9　A relatively contemporary view of what constitutes myth is advanced by Barthes (1979: 109–59).

10　For Gazzaniga's more recent (but essentially unchanged) views on modularity and memory, see Gazzaniga (1985: 100–6).

11　The distinction between personally experienced knowledge and knowledge structured by others, shares aspects in common with Russel's distinction between knowledge by *acquaintance* and knowledge by *description*. (Cf. Russel 1959)

12　Elsewhere we find Gombrich alluding to the relationship between art and language. For example: 'Just as the study of poetry remains incomplete without an awareness of the language of prose, so, I believe, the study of art will be increasingly supplemented by inquiry into the linguistics of the visual image' (1977: 7).

13　Regarding linguistic anchorage, see my reference to Barthes in note 5 of my introduction to this book.

14　Regarding the intention to explicate the representational visual image as being a symptom of the left hemisphere's biologically evolved tendency to dominate in processing information, Michael Youngblood has suggested the following hypothesis to me.

　　Our early ancestors first developed a sophisticated sense of sight. But because mental images of things in the real world could not be transmitted over time and space, vocalization became the means by which early hominids communicated familiar locations in their range. Thus the relationship between verbalizing to others about locations of places in the real world (which were undoubtedly utterances describing the place itself or mental images of it) and the evolution of our contemporary proclivity to vocalize about representational images depicting objects from the real world.

　　Youngblood goes on to propose that although both systems of communication (visual and verbal) are separate entities and occupy principally different locations in the brain, they are inextricably linked to one another via biological evolution. Thus, although a picture may be worth a thousand words, the question is, which thousand do justice to the picture? We will continue to use language to interpret images just as our early ancestors used vocalizations to convey images of locations. There is meaning in the representational image itself just as there is extended meaning in the verbalization of it. (Personal correspondence 1986)

While this hypothesis, which shares features in common with those of Marshack (chapter 3.2), may certainly help to account for why so much is said about the representational visual image, it does not necessarily follow that its meaning is truly *extended* through verbalization. It could be, as I have suggested, that a representation's intuitively (i.e. non-verbal) perceived meaning is simply altered or even distorted by lengthy descriptions. In other words, because certain behaviours may be partially explicable in terms of our biologically evolved tendencies, does not necessarily imply that they are in all instances desirable.

7 A TRANSFORMATIONAL THEORY OF AESTHETICS

1   Levy (1976) and Schweiger (1985) do, however, make connections between neuropsychology and the arts. I review certain psychological and phenomenological theories and relate them to my own theory in chapter 8.

2   I have, of course, substantiated this view in detail and there is therefore no need to reiterate it here.

3   I am contending, therefore, that a certain kind of aesthetic experience is induced by its object, for my purposes, the representational visual image. It is thus not a case of aesthetic experience resulting because of the wilful adoption of a certain mental attitude.

4   This type of understanding is by no means simple but involves complex processes rooted in our experientially and inter-sensorially derived understanding of the phenomenal world. For example, that liquids generally do not resist solids, that wheels are of a certain shape and density, and so forth. See chapter 5.5.

5   My concept of *equivocal reality* perhaps shares aspects in common with Langer's of the *virtual object* and *virtual space*. Cf. Langer 1967.

6   Mandler defines 'mind' and 'mentalism' as follows, 'Briefly, they refer to the view of man as an integrated complex of trans-formational, interpretive, and structural mechanisms. All input is subjected to some transformations – all output is the result of structural mechanisms' (1975: vii–viii).

7   It is also true that the tendency to overtly respond to filmic situations is not confined to parts of France and Italy. At student film society meetings the audience is often seen to gesticulate, shout, and so forth, in response to a film. Although there are clearly strong ritualistic elements involved, the response nonetheless suggests the audience's capacity to relate the passing illusion of film to life values.

8   This conclusion might appear to share aspects in common with Bell's (1914) theory of *significant form*. Bell's argument is essentially that because the forms found in art serve no obviously

practical function, they become significant in that they generate an 'esthetic emotion'. We thus find regarding boat paintings: 'Imagine a boat in complete isolation, detach it from man and his urgent activities and fabulous history, what is it that remains, what is that to which we still react emotionally? What but pure form' (213).

There are, however, marked distinctions between Bell's views and my own. Bell does not acknowledge, as I have done, that representational imagery is first capable of containing life values (a full existential life, etc.) and it is only our suppression of these that can lend an image its extraordinary visual significance.

9   This view clearly shares aspects in common with Langer (1967) when she says: 'the free exercise of artistic intuition often depends on clearing the mind of intellectual prejudice and false conceptions that inhibit people's natural responsiveness' (396). And elsewhere we find:

> If academic training has caused us to think of pictures primarily as examples of schools, periods or the classes that Croce decries ('landscapes', 'portraits', 'interiors', etc.), we are prone to think *about* the picture, gathering quickly all available data for intellectual judgements and so close and clutter the paths of intuitive response.
>
> (Langer 1967: 397)

8   ART AND AESTHETIC EXPERIENCE

1   Elsewhere Diffey has talked at length about the nature of art. See Diffey (1985), for example.
2   Although clear differences exist, Mitias' notion of purposive form may be compared to Bell's (1914) theory of significant form. See chapter 7, note 8, of this book.
3   As Wollheim has suggested, however, there exist certain inconsistencies in Collingwood's overall position. Central to Collingwood's theory of art is the thesis that the work of art does not merely reflect, it is identical with, something initially fully formed in the artist's mind (which in relation to the visual arts we might think of as relating to the mental image). The notion of a fully formed 'mental precursor' to the art work itself is contradicted, however, by the view that the work of art is inseparable from the activity that brings it about (Wollheim 1987: 358 note 8). Diffey has also referred to this inconsistency in Collingwood's thinking (Diffey 1985: 51 note 1).
4   Wollheim notes that the notion of 'thematization' derives from the Prague school of linguists, although there it is used differently.
5   Levy (1976) has developed a neuropsychologically based hypothesis as to why it might be that we tend to perceive pictures left to right.
6   Berleant (1970) argues that: 'If the definition of art is taken

exclusively as a conceptual, analytic problem, independent of the activity of the arts, the discussion dissipates into interminable wrangling that ends with claims for its very impossibility' (155).

7 A fundamental reason for my scepticism is that artists themselves are often unsure of their intentions when creating their works, and even when the work is complete often find difficulty in qualifying its meaning.

8 Although differences may exist between sexually explicit imagery as found in 'men's magazines' and erotic *art*, erotic art is often problematic for the art theoretician or aesthetician. Bullough thus suggests: 'But it is safe to infer that, in art practice, explicit references to organic affections, to the material existence of the body, especially in sexual matters, lie normally below the Distance-limit, and can be touched upon by Art *only with special precautions*' (1983: 73). Regarding the nude in art, Berleant suggests:

> Moreover, the desire for union with another human body has so powerful a place among our basic drives that the nude as an art form is one which cannot and should not suppress erotic feeling. We are more ready now than ever before to recognize the legitimate place of the erotic in art and art in the erotic. Few objects possess such intensity of emotional involvement as does the human body, and it is little wonder that artists constantly find themselves drawn to reveal its endless transformations and to write new variations on this fundamental theme.
>
> (Berleant 1970: 106–7)

Kenneth Clark (1956) has gone so far as to suggest that the nude constitutes an art form in its own right. From a biological/ cognitive perspective, one possible explanation for the peculiar status of the erotic in art is provided by Mandler (1975), who, when referring to emotional states, suggests:

> It could be argued that one of the distinctions we need to make in the discussion of emotional states is, *in this case only*, determined by differential autonomic arousal. Sexual stimuli may thus be considered to differ from other stimuli in that they produce parasympathetic arousal, a specific perceptual syndrome consequent on such arousal, and structures that are specifically related to sexual and lustful emotion.
>
> (Mandler 1975: 241)

9 This view relates to my own, found in my introduction (section 4), when I proposed, 'Given that the human brain is universal and it follows that a greater understanding of its function is relevant to common areas of human activity', etc.

10 Berleant goes on to suggest that this argument suffers from several difficulties. One of these is that questions of art, typically an

afterthought of philosophy, have regularly been approached under the influence of other considerations – moral, metaphysical, epistemological, formal.... 'Indeed it has been customary for philosophers to deal with the theory of art after having already developed a philosophical position, so that their aesthetics becomes a consequence of their position....' One finds this true from Schopenhauer and Nietzsche to Langer and Goodman (93).

11 Berleant's arguments are by no means confined to the representational visual image, however, but include certain contemporary art forms which are so designed as to encourage a personal involvement. I return to this point in section 5.

12 The version referred to here can be found in Coleman (1983: 56–126).

13 There are, however, marked differences between Bullough's concept of Distance and mine of cathectic transference. Bullough thus argues that Distancing initially relates partially to the distancing power of the individual and partially to the nature of the artistic medium (71). Therefore, although he takes into account the possible effects of the medium (its tendency to under- or over-distance), he proposes that these should be wilfully mediated by the Distancing power of the individual. I, on the other hand, have almost exclusively emphasized the potential (aesthetic) effects of the medium form, for my purposes the representational visual image, which automatically generates certain cognitive processes leading to cathectic transference, affective import, and so forth. I return to this distinction when criticizing Bullough's views in section 5.

14 Berleant (1986) suggests that we can also attain experiential unity with the traditional arts and qualifies this view at length in footnotes (96–7). While I have myself argued at length that the traditional art of visual representation can initially generate a certain kind of experiential unity, I have, of course, pointed out that this unity is not ultimately (psychologically) viable because of the communicative constraints of the medium.

9 THE TRANSFORMATIONAL PLANES

1 For Wofflin (1932), who consolidated formal analysis, painterly composition was one of the major sources of aesthetic pleasure. He thus considered that the aesthetician should concentrate on a painting's purely formal visual elements, its forms, lines, colours, contrasts, and textures.

2 The importance of our capacity to tactually verify the nature of an object's spatial relations should not be underestimated, as research by Kennedy (1974, 1977) on the blind has shown.

3 The point here is that the mental processes allowing us to causally link the visual-spatial characteristics of a representation to its

referent do not need to be learned in any formal sense. The
capacity to linguistically link such characteristics does need to be
learned (for example, the capacity to link a certain configuration
to the names *horse, stream, clouds,* etc.). See also chapter 4, note 1.

4   This does not imply that clear criteria exist enabling us to identify a
particular set of images as denoting a 'landscape', for example. It
is nonetheless true to say that the juxtaposition of certain image
forms are generally associated with certain real life situations.
This is evidenced by the fact that when we come across a picture
which confounds the laws of such situations (a 'landscape' by
Magritte, for example), we find the effect incongruous.

5   Whereas the representational plane may inform that certain trees
in *The Hay-Wain* are farther away than others because of our
visually derived knowledge of trees, in principle it cannot inform
that the trees are solid (or the stream is liquid, etc.) The
existential plane does provide this information, however, because
it activates (originally) intersensorially perceived knowledge.

APPENDIX

1   It is fair to point out that Fuller has since partially changed his
views. We thus find him writing more recently:

> For myself, I began to seek a firmer grounding for my ideas
> about art. At first I tried to root aesthetics in psychology and
> biology; *Art and Psychoanalysis*, first published in 1980 ... is
> concerned with such ideas. But I soon found that this way of
> thinking had its limits. Aesthetics could be reduced to neither
> biology nor psychology; and these disciplines could explain
> precious little about the transforming and creative influence of
> a living tradition.
>
> (Fuller 1988: 8)

BIBLIOGRAPHY

Arnheim, R. (1974) *Art and Visual Perception*, Berkeley, CA: University of California Press.

Bakan, P. (1969) 'Hypnotizability, laterality of eye movement and functional brain asymmetry', *Perceptual and Motor Skills* 28: 927–32.

Balonov, L. and Deglin, V. (1977) 'Vosprijatie zvukovyx nerecevyx obrazov (sluxovoj i muzykal'nyj gnozis) v usolovijax inaktivacii domintnogo i nedominant-nogo polusarij', *Fiziologija Celoveka* 3: 415–23.

Barthes, R. (1979) *Mythologies*, Paladin.

—— (1982) *Image-Music-Text*, London: Fontana.

—— (1984) *Camera Lucida*, London: Fontana.

Basser, L. (1962) 'Hemiplegia of early onset and the faculty of speech with special reference to the effects of hemispherectomy', *Brain* 85: 427–60.

Battersby, N., Bender, M., Pollack, M., and Kahn, R. (1956) 'Unilateral spatial agnosia (inattention)', *Brain* 79: 68–75.

Bell, C. (1914) *Art*, London: Chatto & Windus.

Berleant, A. (1970) *The Aesthetic Field*, Springfield, IL: Charles C Thomas.

—— (1986) 'Experience and theory in aesthetics', in M. Mitias (ed.) *Possibility of the Aesthetic Experience*, Dordrecht: Martinus Nijhoff.

Berlyne, D. (1971) *Aesthetics and Psychobiology*, New York: Appleton Century Crofts.

—— (1971) *Studies in New Experimental Aesthetics*, London: Wiley.

Bever, T. (1983) 'Cerebral lateralization, cognitive asymmetry, and human consciousness', in E. Perecman (ed.) *Cognitive Processing in the Right Hemisphere*, New York: Academic Press.

Bever, T. and Chiarello, R. (1974) 'Cerebral dominance in musicians and nonmusicians', *Science* 185: 537–9.

Block, N. (1981) *Imagery*, Cambridge, MA: MIT Press.

Boden, M. (1979) *Piaget*, Brighton: Harvester Press.

Bogen, J. (1969a) 'The other side of the brain. I. Dysgraphia and dyscopia following cerebral commissurotomy', *Bulletin of the Los Angeles Neurological Society* 34: 73–105.

—— (1969b) 'The other side of the brain. II. An oppositional mind',

Bulletin of the Los Angeles Neurological Society 34: 135–62.

Bogen, J. and Vogel, P. (1962) 'Cerebral commissurotomy in man. Preliminary case report', *Bulletin of the Los Angeles Neurological Society* 27: 169.

—— (1963) 'Treatment of generalized seizures by cerebral commissurotomy', *Surgical Forum* 14: 431.

Borod, J. and Caron, H. (1980) 'Facedness and emotion related to lateral dominance, sex and expression type', *Neuropsychologia* 18: 237–41.

Borod, J., Koff, E., and Caron, H. (1983) 'Right hemispheric specialization for the expression and appreciation of emotion: a focus on the face', in E. Perecman (ed.) *Cognitive Processing in the Right Hemisphere*, New York: Academic Press.

Brain, R. (1941) 'Visual disorientation with special reference to the lesions of the right cerebral hemisphere', *Brain* 64: 108–72.

Broca, P. (1861) 'Nouvelle observation d'aphémie produite par une lésion de la moite postérieure des deuxième et troisième circonvolutions frontales', *Bulletin de la Société Anatomique de Paris* 36: 398–407.

Bruce, V. and Green, P. (1987) *Visual Perception*, Hove, Sussex: Lawrence Erlbaum.

Bryden, M. (1982) *Laterality*, New York: Academic Press.

Bryden, M. and Ley, G. (1983) 'Right hemispheric involvement in imagery and affect', in E. Perecman (ed.) *Cognitive Processing in the Right Hemisphere*, New York: Academic Press.

Bullough, E. (1912) '"Psychical distance" as a factor in art and as an aesthetic principle', *British Journal of Psychology* 5: 87–98.

—— (1919) 'The relation of aesthetics to psychology', *British Journal of Psychology* 10: 43–50.

—— (1921) 'Recent work in experimental aesthetics', *British Journal of Aesthetics* 12: 76–99.

—— (1983) 'Aesthetic experience as mental distance', in E. Colman (ed.) *Varieties of Aesthetic Experience*, Lanham: University Press of America.

Buschbaum, M. and Fedio, P. (1970) 'Hemispheric differences in evoked potentials to verbal and nonverbal stimuli on the left and right visual fields', *Physiology and Behavior* 5: 207–10.

Campbell, R. (1978) 'Asymmetries in interpreting and expressing a posed facial expression', *Cortex* 14: 327–42.

Cicone, M., Wapner, W., and Gardner, H. (1980) 'Sensitivity to emotional expressions and situations in organic patients', *Cortex* 16: 154–8.

Clark, K. (1956) *The Nude*, New York: Capricorn Books.

Cohn, R. (1971) 'Differential cerebral processing of noise and verbal stimuli', *Science* 172: 599–601.

Coleman, E. (ed.) (1983) *Varieties of Aesthetic Experience*, Lanham: University Press of America.

Collingwood, R. (1938) *The Principles of Art*, Oxford: Clarendon Press.

Crossley, D. (1975) 'Aesthetic attitude: back in gear with Bullough', *Personalist* 56: 336–45.

Crozier, W. and Chapman, A. (1981) 'Aesthetic preferences: prestige and social class', in D. O'Hare (ed.) *Psychology and the Arts*, Sussex: Harvester Press.

Curry, F. (1967) 'A comparison of left-handed and right-handed subjects on verbal and nonverbal dichotic listening tasks', *Cortex* 3: 343–52.

Danto, A. (1984) 'The artworld', in R. Ross (ed.) *An Anthology of Aesthetic Theory*, Albany: State University of New York.

Day, M. (1964) 'An eye movement phenomenon relating to attention, thought and anxiety', *Perceptual and Motor Skills* 19: 443–6.

De Renzi, E. and Spinnler, H. (1967) 'Impaired performance on colour tasks in patients with hemispheric damage', *Cortex* 3: 194–217.

Deglin, V. (1976) 'Split brain', *Unesco Courier*, January: 5–32.

Dennis, M. and Whitaker, H. (1976) 'Language acquisition following hemi-decortication: linguistic superiority of the left over the right hemisphere', *Brain and Language* 3: 404–43.

Dewey, J. (1934) *Art as Experience*, New York: Mintin, Balch.

Dickie, G. (1974) *Art and the Aesthetic*, Ithaca: Cornell University Press.

Diffey, T. (1985) *Tolstoy's 'What is Art?'*, London: Croom Helm.

—— (1986) 'The idea of aesthetic experience', in M. Mitias (ed.) *Possibility of the Aesthetic Experience*, Dordrecht: Martinus Nijhoff.

Dimond, S. (1978) *Introducing Neuropsychology*, Springfield, IL: Charles C. Thomas.

—— (1979) 'Symmetry and asymmetry in the vertebrate brain', in D. Oakley and H. Plotkin (eds) *Brain, Behaviour and Evolution*, London: Methuen.

Dreyfus, H. (1972) *What Computers Can't Do*, New York: Harper & Row.

Dufrenne, M. (1973) *The Phenomenology of Aesthetic Experience*, Evanston: Northwestern University Press.

Dziemidok, B. (1986) 'Controversy about aesthetic attitude: does aesthetic attitude condition aesthetic experience?' in M. Mitias (ed.) *Possibility of Aesthetic Experience*, Dordrecht: Martinus Nijhoff.

Eccles, J. (1965) The brain and unity of conscious experience, *The 19th Arthur Stanley Eddying Memorial Lecture*, Cambridge: Cambridge University Press.

Eccles, J. (1980) *The Human Psyche*, Berlin: Springer Verlag.

Eco, U. (1976) *A Theory of Semiotics*, Bloomington: Indiana University Press.

Ehrlichman, H. and Weinberger, A. (1979) 'Lateral eye movements and hemispheric asymmetry: a critical review', *Psychological Bulletin* 85: 1080–101.

Eng, H. (1966) *The Psychology of Children's Drawing*, London: Routledge & Kegan Paul.

Entus, A. (1977) 'Hemispheric asymmetry in processing dichotically presented speech and nonspeech stimuli by infants', in S. Segalowitz and F. Gruber (eds) *Language Development and Neurological Theory*,

New York: Harper & Row.

Eysenck, H. (1981) 'Aesthetic preferences and individual differences', in D. O'Hare (ed.) *Psychology and the Arts*, Brighton: Harvester Press.

Festinger, F. (1957) *A Theory of Cognitive Dissonance*, New York: Harper & Row.

Fisher, E., Bogen, J., and Vogel, P. (1965) 'Cerebral commissurotomy: a second case report', *Journal of American Medical Association* 194: 1328–9.

Fodor, J. (1983) *The Modularity of Mind*, Cambridge, MA: MIT Press.

Freeman, N. (1980) *Strategies of Representation in Young Children. Analysis of Spatial Skills and Drawing Processes*, London: Academic Press.

Fuller, P. (1981) *Art and Psychoanalysis*, London: Writers & Readers.

—— (1983a) *The Naked Artist*, London: Writers & Readers.

—— (1983b) *Aesthetics After Modernism*, London: Writers & Readers.

—— (1988) *Seeing Through Berger*, London: Claridge Press.

Gaede, S., Parson, O. and Bertera, J. (1978) 'Hemispheric differences in music perception: aptitude vs. experience', *Neuropsychologia* 7: 195–204.

Galaburda, M., LeMay M., Kempter, T., and Geschwind, N. (1978) 'Right-left asymmetries in the brain', *Science* 199: 852–6.

Galin, D. and Ornstein, K. (1972) 'Lateral specialization of cognitive mode: an EEG study', *Psychophysiology* 9: 412–18.

Gardner, H. (1975) *The Shattered Mind*, New York: Knorf.

—— (1981) 'Children's perceptions of works of art: a developmental portrait', in D. O'Hare (ed.) *Psychology and the Arts*, Brighton: Harvester Press.

—— (1984) *Frames of Mind*, London: William Heinemann.

Gardner, H., Brownwell, H., Wapner, W., and Michelow, D. (1983) 'Missing the point: the role of the right hemisphere in processing of complex linguistic materials', in E. Perecman (ed.) *Cognitive Processing in the Right Hemisphere*, New York: Academic Press.

Gazzaniga, M. (1970) *The Bisected Brain*, New York: Appleton-Century Crofts.

—— (1985) *The Social Brain*, New York: Basic Books Inc.

Gazzaniga, M. and Hillyard, S. (1971) 'Language and speech capacity of the right hemisphere', *Neuropsychologia* 9: 273–80.

Gazzaniga, M. and LeDoux, J. (1978) *The Integrated Mind*, New York: Plenum Press.

Geschwind, N. (1974) *Selected Papers on Language and the Brain* 1, Dordrecht: D. Reidel.

—— (1976) 'Approach to a theory of localization of emotion in the human brain', paper presented at International Neuropsychological Symposium, Rob-Amadour, France.

Gibson, J. (1968) *The Senses Considered as Perceptual Systems*, London: Allen & Unwin.

Goldstein, K. (1963) *Human Nature in the Light of Psychopathology*, New York: Schocken Books.

Gombrich, E. (1967) *The Story of Art*, London: Phaidon.

—— (1977) *Art and Illusion*, London: Phaidon.
—— (1978) *Meditations on a Hobby Horse*, London: Phaidon.
—— (1979) *Ideals and Idols*, London: Phaidon.
—— (1982) *The Image and the Eye*, London: Phaidon.
Goodman, N. (1968) *The Languages of Art*, New York: Bobbs-Merrill.
Goodnow, J. (1977) *Children's Drawing*, London: Open Books.
Gordon, H. (1980) 'Right hemisphere comprehension of verbs in patients with complete forebrain commissurotomy: use of the dichotic method and manual performance', *Brain and Language* 11: 76–86.
Gur, R. and Gur, R. (1977a) 'Correlates of conjugate lateral eye movements in man', in Harnard *et al.* (eds) *Lateralization of the Nervous System*, New York: Academic Press.
—— (1977b) 'Sex differences in the relations among handedness. Sighting dominance and eye-acuity', *Neuropsychologia* 15: 585–90.
Hall, M., Hall, G., and Lavoie, P. (1968) 'Ideation in patients with unilateral or bilateral midline brain lesions', *Journal of Abnormal Psychology* 73: 526–31.
Hamylin, D. (1978) *Experience and Growth of Understanding*, London: Routledge & Kegan Paul.
Hartline, H. (1942) *The Neural Mechanisms of Vision*, The Harvey Lectures, 1941–2, Series 37, 39–68, London.
Hecaen, J. and Angelergues, R. (1962) 'Agnosia for faces', *Archives of Neurology* 1: 92–100.
Hecaen, J. and Sauguet, J. (1971) 'Cerebral dominance in left-handed subjects', *Cortex* 7: 19–48.
Hochberg, J. and Brooks, V. (1962) 'Pictorial recognition as an unlearned ability', *American Journal of Psychology* 75: 624–8.
Hogg, J. (1969) *Psychology and the Visual Arts*, Harmondsworth: Penguin.
Hohmann, G. (1966) 'Some effects of spinal cord lesions on experienced emotional feelings', *Psychophysiology* 3: 143–56.
Hookway, C. (1984) *Minds, Machines and Mechanisms*, Cambridge: Cambridge University Press.
Hospers, J. (1976) *Meaning and Truth in the Arts*, Chapel Hill: University of North Carolina Press.
—— (1982) *Understanding the Arts*, Englewood Cliffs: Prentice-Hall.
Hubel, D. and Wiesel, T. (1959) 'Receptive fields of single neurons in the cat's striate cortex', *Journal of Physiology* 148: 574–91.
Ingarden, R. (1973) *The Cognition of the Literary Work of Art*, Evanston: Northwestern University Press.
Jackson, J. (1874) 'On the nature of duality of the brain', *Medical Press Circular* 1: 19.
Jakobson, R. (1980) *Brain and Language*, Columbus, OH: Slavica Publishers.
Kant, I. (1790, 1914) *Kant's Critique of Judgement*, London: Macmillan and Co. Ltd.
Kennedy, J. (1974) *A Psychology of Picture Perception*, San Francisco: Jossey-Bass Publishers.

—— (1977) 'Pictures to see and pictures to touch', in D. Perkins and B. Leondar (eds) *The Arts and Cognition*, Baltimore: The Johns Hopkins University Press.

Kimura, D. (1961a) 'Some effects of temporal lobe damage on auditory perception', *Canadian Journal of Psychology* 167: 156–65.

—— (1961b) 'Cerebral dominance and perception of verbal stimuli', *Canadian Journal of Psychology* 15: 166–71.

—— (1963) 'Right temporal lobe damage: perception of unfamiliar stimuli after damage', *Archives of Neurology* 8: 264–71.

—— (1964) 'Left-right differences in the perception of melodies', *Quarterly Journal of Experimental Psychology* 16: 355–8.

—— (1967) 'Functional asymmetry of the brain in dichotic listening', *Cortex* 3: 163–78.

Kimura, D. and Archibald, Y. (1974) 'Motor functions of the left hemisphere', *Brain* 97: 337–50.

Kimura, D. and Folb, S. (1968) 'Neural processing in backwards speech sounds', *Science* 161: 395–6.

King, F. and Kimura, D. (1972) 'Left-ear superiority in dichotic perception of vocal nonverbal sounds', *Canadian Journal of Psychology* 26: 111–16.

Kinsbourne, M. (1975) 'The ontogeny of cerebral dominance', in D. Aaronson and R. Rieber (eds) *Developmental Psycholinguistics and Communication Disorders*, New York: New York Academy of Sciences.

—— (1978) 'Evolution of language in relation to lateralization', in M. Kinsbourne (ed.) *Asymmetrical Function of the Brain*, Cambridge: Cambridge University Press.

Knox, C. and Kimura, D. (1970) 'Cerebral processing of nonverbal sounds in boys and girls', *Neuropsychologia* 8: 227–37.

Korzenik, D. (1977) 'Saying it with pictures', in D. Perkins and B. Leondar (eds) *The Arts and Cognition*, Baltimore: The Johns Hopkins University Press.

Langer, S. (1967) *Feeling and Form*, London: Routledge & Kegan Paul.

—— (1977) 'Art and symbolic expression', in G. Dickie and R. Scalfani (eds) *Aesthetics*, London: St Martin's Press.

Lassen, N. and Ingvar, D. (1972) 'Radioisotopic assessment of regional cerebral blood flows', *Progress in Nuclear Medicine* 1, Baltimore: University Park Press.

LeDoux, J., Wilson, D., and Gazzaniga, M. (1977a) 'A divided mind: observations on the conscious properties of the separated hemispheres', *Annals of Neurology* 2: 417–21.

LeDoux, J., Risse, G., Springer, S., Wilson, D., and Gazzaniga, M. (1977b) 'Cognition and commissurotomy', *Brain* 100: 87–104.

Lennenberg, E. (1967) *Biological Foundations of Language*, New York: Wiley.

Lessing, G. (1984) *Laocoon*, Baltimore: The Johns Hopkins University Press.

Lettvin, J. (1959) 'What the frog's eye tells the frog's brain', in P. Dodwell (ed.) *Perceptual Processing: Stimulus Equivalence and Pattern*

Recognition, New York: Appleton Century Crofts.

Levi-Agresti, J. and Sperry, R. (1968) 'Differential perceptual capacities in major and minor hemispheres', *proceedings of the National Academy of Science USA* 61: 1151.

Levy, J. (1969) 'Possible basis for the evolution of lateral specialization of the human brain', *Nature* (London) 214, 614–15.

—— (1974) 'Psychobiological implications of bilateral asymmetry', in S. Dimond and J. Beaumont (eds) *Hemispheric Function in the Human Brain*, London: Elek Science.

—— (1976) 'Lateral dominance and aesthetic preference', *Neuropsychologia* 14: 431–45.

Levy, J., Trevarthen, C., and Sperry, R. (1972) 'Perception of bilateral chimeric studies following hemispheric deconnection', *Brain* 95: 61–8.

Ley, R. (1982) 'Cerebral laterality and imagery', in A. Scheikh (ed.) *Imagery: Current Theory, Research and Application*, New York: Wiley.

Ley, R. and Bryden, M. (1979) 'Hemispheric differences in recognizing faces and emotions', *Brain and Language* 7: 127–38.

Lindauer, M. (1981) 'Aesthetic experience: a neglected topic in the psychology of the arts', in D. O'Hare (ed.) *Psychology and the Arts*, Brighton: Harvester Press.

Lindsay, P. and Norman, D. (1977) *Human Information Processing: An Introduction to Psychology*, New York: Academic Press.

Lipps, T. (1960) 'Empathy and Abstraction', in M. Rader (ed.) *A Modern Book of Esthetics*, Fort Worth: Holt, Rinehart & Winston.

Luquet, G. (1913) *Les Dessins d'un Enfant*, Paris: Alcan.

—— (1927) *Le Dessin Enfantin*, Paris: Alcan.

Mackay, D. (1972) Personal communication to Michael Gazzaniga, cited in M. Gazzaniga, 'One brain – two minds?' *American Science* 60, 311–17.

Mandler, G. (1975) *Mind and Emotion*, New York: Wiley.

—— (1985) *Cognitive Psychology*, New Jersey: Lawrence Erlbaum Associates.

Marr, D. (1982) *Vision: A Computational Investigation into the Human Representation and Processing of Information*, Oxford: W.H. Freeman & Company.

Marshack, A. (1972) 'Cognitive aspects of upper paleolithic engraving', *Current Anthropology* 13: 455–77.

—— (1976) 'Some implications of the paleolithic symbol evidence for the origins of language', *Current Anthropology* 17: 274–82.

Merleau-Ponty, M. (1962) *Phenomenology of Perception*, London: Routledge & Kegan Paul.

—— (1964) *The Primacy of Perception*, Evanston: Northwestern University Press.

Metz, C. (1982) *Psychoanalysis and the Cinema*, London: Macmillan Press.

Miller, G., Galenter, E., and Pribram, K. (1960) *Plans and the Structure of Behavior*, New York: Holt Langer.

Milner, B. and Taylor, L. (1972) 'Right hemisphere superiority in tactile pattern recognition after cerebral commissurotomy: evidence for nonverbal memory', *Neuropsychologia* 10: 1–10.

Milner, B., Taylor, L., and Sperry, R. (1968) 'Lateralized suppression of dichotically presented digits after commissural section in man', *Science* 161: 184–5.

Mitias, M. (1986) 'Can we speak of "aesthetic experience"?', in M. Mitias (ed.) *Possibility of the Aesthetic Experience*, Dordrecht: Martinus Nijhoff.

Molfese, D. (1977) 'Infant cerebral asymmetry', in S. Segalowitz and F. Gruber (eds) *Language Development and Neurological Theory*, New York: Academic Press.

Molfese, D., Freeman, R., and Palermo, D. (1975) 'The ontogeny of brain lateralization for speech and nonspeech stimuli', *Brain and Language* 2: 356–68.

Moscovitch, M. and Olds, J. (1982) 'Asymmetries in spontaneous facial expression and their possible relation to hemispheric specialization', *Neuropsychologia* 20: 71–81.

Myers, R. (1956) 'Function of corpus callosum in interlocular transfer', *Brain* 79: 358–63.

Nadel, S. (1937) 'A field experiment in racial psychology', *British Journal of Psychology* 28: 195–211.

Nagel, T. (1971) 'Brain bisection and the unity of consciousness', *Synthese* 22: 396–413.

Nebes, R. (1972) 'Dominance in the minor hemisphere in commissurotomized man on a test of figural unification', *Brain* 95: 633–88.

—— (1973) 'Perception of spatial relationships by the right and left hemispheres of commissurotomized man', *Neuropsychologia* 11: 358–63.

Needham, C. (1982) *The Principles of Cerebral Dominance*, Springfield, IL: Charles C Thomas.

Nunally, J. (1977) 'Meaning-processing and rated pleasantness', *Scientific Aesthetics* 1: 168–81.

Osborne, H. (1970) *The Art of Appreciation*, Oxford: Oxford University Press.

Panofsky, E. (1955) *Meaning in the Visual Arts*, New York: Doubleday Anchor.

—— (1968) *Idea: A Concept in Art Theory*, Columbia: University of South Carolina Press.

Pateman, T. (1980) *Language Truth and Politics*, Lewes: Stroud.

—— (1983) 'How is understanding an advertisement possible?', in H. Davis and P. Walton (eds) *Language Image Media*, Oxford: Blackwell.

—— (1984a) 'Déjà lu', London: *Times Educational Supplement* (21 December 1984).

—— (1984b) 'On art and things that go bump in the night', unpublished paper delivered at Derbyshire College of Higher Education.

—— (1985) 'Using and defending cognitive theory', in N. Gilbert and C. Heath (eds) *Social Action and Artificial Intelligence*, London: Gower Press.

—— (1986) 'Transparent and translucent icons', *British Journal of Aesthetics* 26, 4.

Peirce, C. (1940) *The Philosophy of Peirce*, London: Routledge & Kegan Paul.

Perecman, E. (1983) 'Discovering buried treasure – a look at the cognitive potential of the right hemisphere', in E. Perecman (ed.) *Cognitive Processing in the Right Hemisphere*, New York: Academic Press.

Perkins, D. and Leondar, B. (1977) 'Introduction – a cognitive approach to the arts', in D. Perkins and B. Leondar (eds) *The Arts and Cognition*, Baltimore: The Johns Hopkins University Press.

Piaget, J. (1966) *The Origins of Intelligence in the Child*, London: Routledge & Kegan Paul.

—— (1977) *The Child's Conception of the World*, London: Routledge & Kegan Paul.

Piaget, J. and Inhelder, B. (1956) *The Child's Conception of Space*, London: Routledge & Kegan Paul.

—— (1969) *The Psychology of the Child*, London: Routledge & Kegan Paul.

—— (1971) *Mental Imagery in the Child*, London: Routledge & Kegan Paul.

Pucetti, R. (1973) 'Brain bisection and personal identity', *British Journal for the Philosophy of Science* 24: 339–55.

—— (1976) 'The mute self: a reaction to De Witt's alternative account of the split-brain data', *British Journal for the Philosophy of Science* 27: 65–73.

Rasmussen, T. and Milner, B. (1977) 'The role of early infant left-brain injury in determining lateralization of cerebral speech functions', in S. Dimond and B. Blizzard (eds) *Evolution and Lateralization of the Brain*, New York: New York Academy of Sciences.

Risse, G., LeDoux, J., Springer, S., Wilson, D., and Gazzaniga, M. (1977) 'The anterior commissure in man: functional variation in a multi-sensory system', *Neuropsychologia* 16: 23–31.

Rosenfield, I. (1985) A hero of the brain, *New York Review*, November: 49–55.

Rosenweig, M. (1951) 'Representation of the two ears at the auditory cortex', *American Journal of Physiology* 167: 147–58.

Ross, E. and Mesulam, M. (1979) 'Dominant language functions of the right hemisphere: prosody and emotional gesturing', *Archives of Neurology* 36: 144–8.

Russel, B. (1959) *The Problems of Philosophy*, Oxford: Oxford University Press.

Sartre, J. (1948) *Psychology of the Imagination*, New York: Philosophical Library.

Saussure, F. (1983) *Course in General Linguistics* (eds) C. Bally and A. Sechehaye, London: Duckworth.

Scruton, R. (1983) *The Aesthetic Understanding*, Manchester: Carcanet.

Schwartz, G., Davidson, R. and Maer, F. (1975) 'Right hemisphere lateralization for emotion in the human brain: interaction with cognition', *Science* 190: 286–8.

Schweiger, A. (1985) 'Harmony of the spheres and hemispheres: the arts and hemispheric specialization', in D. Benson and E. Zaidel (eds) *The Dual Brain*, New York: Guildform Press.

Selfe, L. (1977) *Nadia – A Case of Extraordinary Drawing Ability in Children*, London: Academic Press.

—— (1983) *Normal and Anomalous Representational Drawing Ability in Children*, London: Academic Press.

—— (1985) 'Anomalous drawing development: some clinical studies', in N. Freeman and B. Cox (eds) *Visual Order*, Cambridge: Cambridge University Press.

Semmes, J., Weinstein, S., Ghent, L., and Teuber, H. (1955) 'Spatial orientation in man after cerebral injury: analyses by locus of lesion', *Journal of Psychology* 39, 227–44.

Sontag, S. (1979) *On Photography*, London: Allen Lane.

Sperry, R. (1959) 'Preservation of higher order function in isolated somatic cortex in callosum sectioned cat', *Journal of Neurophysiology* 22: 78.

—— (1964a) 'Problems outstanding in the evolution of brain function', *James Arthur Lecture*, New York: American Museum of Natural History.

—— (1964b) 'The great cerebral commissure', *Scientific American* 210: 42–52.

—— (1966) 'Hemispheric interaction and the mid-brain problem', in J. Eccles (ed.) *Brain and Conscious Experience*, Berlin: Springer-Verlag.

—— (1968) 'Mental unity following surgical disconnection of the cerebral hemispheres', *The Harvey Lecture Series* 62: 293–323.

—— (1979) 'Consciousness, free will and personal identity', in D. Oakley and H. Plotkin (eds) *Brain, Behaviour and Evolution*, London: Methuen.

—— (1982) 'Some effects of disconnecting the cerebral hemispheres', *Science* 217: September, 1223–6.

—— (1983) *Science and Moral Priority*, Oxford: Blackwell.

Sperry, R., Zaidel, E., and Zaidel, D. (1979) 'Self recognition and social awareness in the deconnected hemisphere', *Neuropsychologia*, 17: 153–66.

Springer, S. and Deutsch, G. (1981) *Left Brain, Right Brain*, San Francisco: W.H. Freeman.

Springer, S. and Gazzaniga, M. (1975) 'Dichotic listening in partial and complete split brain patients', *Neuropsychologia* 13: 341–6.

Steele Russel, I. (1979) 'Brain size and intelligence: a comparative perspective', in D. Oakley and H. Plotkin (eds) *Brain, Behaviour and Evolution*, London: Methuen.

Steinberg, S. (1953) 'The eye is a part of the mind', *Partisan Review* 20: 194–212.

Stephan, M. (1988) 'The theatrical Rothko', in P. Abbs and T. Pateman (eds) *Responses to Rothko*, Falmer: University of Sussex, internal publication.

Stolnitz, J. (1960) *Aesthetics and Philosophy of Art Criticism*, Boston:

Houghton Mifflin Company.
—— (1986) 'The actualities of non-aesthetic experience', in M. Mitias (ed.) *Possibility of Aesthetic Experience*, Dordrecht: Martinus Nijhoff.
Thatcher, R., McAlaster, R., Lester., M., Horst, R., and Cantor, D. (1983) 'Hemispheric EEG asymmetries related to cognitive functioning in children', in E. Perecman (ed.) *Cognitive Processing in the Right Hemisphere*, New York: Academic Press.
Turkewitz, G. (1977) 'The development of lateral differentiation in the human infant', *Annals of New York Academy of Sciences* 299: 309–18.
Wada, J. and Davis, A. (1977) 'Fundamental nature of human infant's brain asymmetry', *Canadian Journal of Neurological Sciences* 4, 203–7.
Wada, J. and Rasmussen, T. (1960) 'Intercartoid injection of sodium amytal for the lateralization of cerebral speech dominance: experimental and critical observations', *Journal of Neurosurgery* 17: 152–64.
Warrington, E. and Taylor, M. (1973) 'The contribution of the right parietal lobe to object recognition', *Cortex* 9: 152–64.
—— (1978) 'Two categorical stages of object recognition', *Perception* 7: 203–7.
Weisenberg, T. and McBride, K. (1935) *Aphasia: a clinical and psychological study*, New York: Commonwealth Fund.
Winnicott, D. (1971) *Playing and Reality*, London: Tavistock Publications.
Witelson, S. (1977) 'Early hemisphere specialization and interhemispheric plasticity', in S. Segalowitz and F. Gruber (eds) *Language Development and Neurological Theory*, New York: Academic Press.
Wittgenstein, L. (1921) *Tractatus Logico-Philosophicus*, London: Routledge & Kegan Paul.
Wofflin, H. (1932) *Principles of Art History: The Problem of the Development of Style in Later Art*, New York: Dover Publications.
Wollheim, R. (1968) *Art and its Objects*, London: Harper & Row.
—— (1987) *Painting as an Art*, London: Thames & Hudson.
Yakolev, P. and LeCours, A. (1967) 'The myelogenic cycles of regional maturation of the brain', in A. Minkowski (ed.) *Regional Development of the Brain in Early Life*, Oxford: Blackwell.
Youngblood, M. (1979) 'The hemispherality wagon leaves laterality station at 12.45 for art superiority land', *Studies in Art Education* 21/1: 44–9.
Zaidel, E. (1975) 'A technique for presenting lateralized visual input with prolonged exposure', *Vision Research* 15: 283–9.

INDEX

The
OS X Mavericks
PocketGuide

Jeff**Carlson**

Ginormous knowledge, pocket sized.

201390259

The OS X Mavericks Pocket Guide
Jeff Carlson

Peachpit Press

Find us on the web at www.peachpit.com
To report errors, please send a note to errata@peachpit.com

Peachpit Press is a division of Pearson Education.

Project editor: Clifford Colby
Copyeditor: Scout Festa
Production editor: Katerina Malone
Compositor: Jeff Carlson
Indexer: Valerie Haynes Perry
Cover design: Peachpit Press
Interior design: Peachpit Press

ISBN-13:   9780321961136
ISBN-10:   0321961137

9 8 7 6 5 4 3 2 1

Printed and bound in the United States of America